Barefoot
On Coral Calcium

"AN ELIXIR OF LIFE"
Health Secrets of the Coral of Okinawa

By

Robert R. Barefoot

Forward By
Scott Miller — The Mineral Man

Barefoot on Coral Calcium
An Elixir of Life

This publication is intended to direct the attention of both physician and patient to scientific research being carried out on the significance of calcium supplements to health and to the concept that coral calcium from Okinawa is the best form of supplemental calcium in the opinion of Barefoot. It is for educational purposes. It is not intended to replace the orthodox physician-patient relationship. If you are sick, you are advised to consult a physician, and together, along with your newly gained knowledge from this book, work towards the resolution of your illness.

Preliminary

The Re-Growth of the Coral Reefs of the World

The first time that I ever went to Hawaii, I went swimming off the beach at Waikiki. It was breathtaking! Hundreds of colorful fish were swimming all around me, and I was floating over the most beautiful coral imaginable. I was mesmerized. I had not realized that there was such a beautiful place on Earth. The experience remains with me, and every time I think of coral, I think of Hawaii and the most beautiful ocean on Earth. Ironically, a few decades later I would learn that not only does the coral make the oceans clean and pristine, but some coral when eaten can have almost magical curative power. Currently, I am known by many as the "King of Coral Calcium."

Thus, I have a passionate interest in preserving the coral reefs of the world. The harvesting of the coral calcium is done from the deep open ocean trenches many miles from the coral reefs which are protected by the Japanese Government and the people of Okinawa. However, every time a pound of coral is consumed, I worry about replacement, even though more coral calcium is produced naturally by the oceans than can possibly be consumed. The problem is that the coral reefs are super sensitive and just mild changes in temperature or salinity and run off pollution can destroy them. Over the past decade, more than 30% of the world's coral reefs have been destroyed. The world is obviously facing a crisis. What can be done?

Because of my passion for the coral reefs, I was recently contacted by a representative of the "Russian Academy of Science" Apparently, over the past decade they have perfected a process to re-grow coral reefs at a rapid rate. The technology is currently being held in limbo, waiting for someone to exploit it.

The Russian technology uses a coral ball made of porous concrete specially formulated to induce the rapid growth of coral reefs. Just one month in any ocean water and coral is growing profusely from the ball. Imagine if you live in Los Angeles and could go down to the beach to swim in the new coral reefs in clean and pristine water. The same will one day be true for all oceanside cities all over the world.

Currently, technicians are being trained and the bugs are being removed from the production technology. A new and improved world awaits, but first the public has to get behind the technology. Just imagine not only being involved in curing humanity, but also in curing the oceans. A more noble cause has never before existed. Bob Barefoot intends to make the re-growth of the world's coral reefs his goal, and hopes that many of you will do the same. Let's remove the horror, pain and suffering that degenerative disease causes humanity. Let's cure humanity, and let's grow coral reefs all over the world. Let's cure the oceans.

Plea for Help !!!

Please join Bob Barefoot in supporting the re-growth of the world's coral reefs. Let's cure humanity, let's cure the oceans Go to : "Barefootscureamerica.com"

Barefoot On Coral Calcium

This book is novel, new, controversial and thought-provoking. Based on thirty years of personal research, Robert R. Barefoot, a renowned chemist, presents a powerful argument for the wide-ranging health benefits of marine coral minerals (coral calcium) from Okinawa, Japan. Steeped in mystery, folklore, credible testimonials and emerging science, this book describes how coral remnants collected from the Okinawan ocean floor provide a powerhouse of vital micronutrients and other components. This book focuses on the potent and versatile health benefits of coral minerals and calcium from Okinawa, Japan, when they are used as a dietary supplement. If you are sick, you are advised to consult a physician, and together, along with your newly gained knowledge, work towards the resolution of your illness.

Referred to as "an elixir of life," Barefoot "stands on coral calcium" as the longevity factor that accounts for the robust health and long life of the inhabitants of Okinawa, pointing out that Japanese scientists themselves concluded that the good health and longevity of the inhabitants of Okinawa was due to the "calcium rich coral water" they consume. Barefoot, who has been the champion of calcium health supplements (read his book *The Calcium Factor*) brings coral minerals to the attention of Western society for their potential health benefits as a food supplement. While acknowledging an incomplete understanding of how coral exerts its benefits on health, Barefoot points to the massive amount of literature by the medical research community citing the health benefits of calcium. He also points to the fact that the FDA has on its docket for approval the fact that calcium supplements help to reduce and prevent "various cancers, (#2004Q-0097)," "kidney/urinary stones, (#2004Q-0102)," "hypertension or blood pressure, (#2004Q-0098)," "bone fractures, (#2004Q-0100)," and "menstrual disorders, (#2004Q-0099)." Therefore, if the coral calcium from Okinawa is as Barefoot believes, the best form of supplemental calcium, then those taking it can receive all of the health benefits that the FDA attributes to calcium supplements, and many, many more. This is probably the reason why coral calcium from Okinawa has been consumed for hundreds of years by millions of people. Thus, in the face of controversy in conventional medicine by the doubting Thomas', no controversy exists in Barefoot's mind on the health benefits of marine coral minerals.

Since 1982, Barefoot has watched as nutritional therapy was used to help people cure themselves of diseases when ""doctors said that there was no hope. The truth being was that there was no hope as long as conventional medicine was applied, as pharmaceutical drugs have never cured any degenerative disease. But, God made the human body miraculous so that if it gets what it needs, it can cure itself. And, what the body needs is, not the white chemical killer drugs, but rather it needs only God's natural nutrition. The DNA in our bodies allows us to replicate damaged body parts, but the DNA only works when smothered in calcium, something doctors would rarely recommend. The scientific community, on the other hand, has produced thousands of documents extolling calcium's ability to alter disease. Thus, the only hope to reverse the deadly course modern medicine has put mankind on is to begin the use of God's nutritional therapy.

4

Barefoot on Coral Calcium
An Elixer of Life

The Health Secrets of the Coral of Okinawa.
By
Robert R. Barefoot
Published By:
Pan American International Nutrition Ltd. Publishing
Post Office Box 21389
Wickenburg, AZ 85358 U.S.A.

Pan American International Nutrition Ltd. Publishing
P.O. Box 21389
Wickenburg, AZ 85358

Library of Congress Cataloging in Publication Data
Barefoot, Robert R.
Barefoot on Coral Calcium An Elixir of Life by Robert R. Barefoot -2nd Edition
Bibliography
Includes subjects:

1. Minerals and Longevity
2. Nutritional Medicine
3. Alternative Medicine
4. Coral Calcium
5. Health and Marine Coral

This book was not written to endorse the use of specific products or for any treatment purpose. The conclusions in this book represent the author's opinion of medical, scientific, folkloric and lay writings on the various topics discussed.

ISBN 978-0-9714224-1-4
Printed in the United States

Table of Contents

Endorsements

"Mr. Barefoot is one of the Nation's top Nutritional Therapists, a chemist, scientist in the fields of biochemistry, hydrocarbon extraction and metal extraction from ores, inventor and holder of numerous patents, public speaker, writer, and outstanding business entrepreneur, a man of great integrity, enthusiasm, determination, loyalty, and tireless energy, coupledwith a great personality. Mr. Barefoot has achieved wideacclaim in recent years for his biochemistry research into the interrelationship between disease and malnutrition, espousingthat degenerative diseases are caused by mineral and vitamin deficiencies," Howard W. Pollock, Congressman (Alaska) Retired, Past President Safari Club International, Ducks Unlimited, and The National Rifle Association.

"I have been a practicing physician for the past 25 years. I am a fellow of the American College of OB-GYN and a diplomat of the American Board of OB-GYN. Mr. Barefoot has helped me immensely to understand the complex chemistry of how calcium and other minerals contribute to overall health and preventive medicine. I personally know of many individuals who are much healthier today because of Mr. Barefoot's nutritional advice, including myself." Wayne Weber M.D., Family Planning Associates Medical Group Inc., Los Angeles, California.

"I am a heart surgeon at Westchester Medical Center in Valhalla, New York, one of the largest open-heart surgery centers in the United States. I have had a special interest in nutrition over the past 30 years and have lectured on this

subject throughout the United States, particularly its relationship to heart disease and other degenerative diseases. It is in this capacity that I have come to know and respect Robert Barefoot. He is an internationally known chemist with numerous international patents. His use of bio-chemistry in the field of hydrocarbon extraction and the field of metal extraction of ores led him to pursue a different line of research over the past two decades, elucidating the intimate relationship between nutrition and disease." Richard W. Pooley, Professor of Surgery, New York Medical College, New York.

"I am a physician, President and Executive Medical Director of Health Insight, S.B.S. and Health Advocate Inc., in the state of Michigan. I have extensive credentials and honors that reach the White House and Heads of States in other countries. Mr. Robert Barefoot is a remarkable gentleman and a scholar who works endlessly to complete his mission to cure America. He has worked over the past 20 years with many medical doctors and scientists across the United States and in other countries doing Orthomolecular Research on various diseases. The information has been culminated in two books, "The Calcium Factor" and "Death by Diet" which have been used technically as Bibles of Nutrition. Many people I know have thanked Mr. Barefoot for both saving their lives and returning them to good health. Mr. Barefoot is an amazing and extraordinary man who is on a 'Great Mission' for all mankind. I thank God for Robert Barefoot." Liska M. Cooper, M.D., Detroit, Michigan.

"I am a physician practicing at the Molecular/Biological level for over 25 years. I lecture extensively in the nutritional medical field in Canada, the United States and internationally. I have attended hundreds of lectures and seminars covering the aspects of medicine including a number of those given by

Robert Barefoot whose discourses easily classify as absolutely excellent! Personal conversations with this man, a highly moral and ethical person, have served to confirm his unusual knowledge in the field of biologically applied nutrition and immunity enhancement." C.T. Taylor, M.D., L.M.C.C., P. Eng., Stony Plain, Alberta.

"I have been an attorney involved in very complex litigation involving natural supplements and their ability to treat or cure various types of illnesses, including cancer. I am well known in Maryland as a litigator, repeatedly being named as one of the outstanding trial attorneys, specializing in complex matters of all natures and have written concerning trial techniques. Mr. Barefoot was engaged as an expert in the use of natural supplements, specifically minerals, and their effect on various forms of cancers. He is a renowned author in this field. There have been many occasions when I found him to be extraordinarily knowledgeable in this field of expertise. My professional opinion is that Mr. Barefoot's knowledge and experience with minerals and other natural substances and their application for the treatment of illnesses is quite unique. In fact, I am not aware of any other individual who possesses the knowledge and expertise in this very important and expanding field as Mr. Barefoot." David Freishtat, Attorney, Freishtat & Sandler, Baltimore, Maryland.

"Mr. Barefoot has been, and continues to be, an advocate for health and natural healing through nutrition and knowledge. He has championed the cause of well over 440,000 American women and children who have been exposed to the toxic effects of silicone implanted devices. Mr. Barefoot, one of the rare silica chemists in the world, has delivered a message of hope to these suffering individuals, who didn't have any hope

*before, but are now arming themselves with the books "**The Calcium Factor**" and "**Death By Diet**" and are spreading the word. The name Barefoot has become a household word. In the past three years, he has traveled to countless meetings and medical conferences throughout the country without charging for his services. Robert Barefoot is a humanitarian and his efforts to educate through his books, informational tapes, lectures and vast media appearances has set a standard of excellence that is well above the norm. His work with hundreds of scientists and medical doctors, researching diet, has elevated him to one of the top speakers on nutrition in the nation."* Jill M. Wood, President Idaho Breast Implant Information Group, Boise Idaho.

*"I recently retired as President and CEO of Bioflora International Inc., a manufacturer of nutritional supplements, liquid mineral extracts, and liquid organic plant foods. I oversaw the formulation and production of what is considered the world's best selling mineral supplement. I was originally introduced to and very impressed by the work of Robert Barefoot, specifically "**The Calcium Factor**" in 1996 but was not afforded the pleasure of a personal introduction until 1998. By that time he had developed a reputation and a title, "The King of Calcium."* G. Scott Miller Past President & CEO, Bioflora Phoenix, Arizona

"I graduated from Harvard University in 1942 (BSC Chemistry) and worked as a Research Director and in corporate management for Franklin Electronics Inc., and have been awarded two patents. Mr. Barefoot has been highly influential in my survival of prostate cancer, with which I was diagnosed in the fall of 1991. Because of his detailed knowledge of biochemistry, he has much more

penetrating knowledge of the relationship between disease and nutrition, a knowledge not available to many trained dieticians because of their lack of biochemical background. With his expertise, he has aided me in not only arresting the progression of my disease, cancer, through diet and nutrition, but also reversing it. Mr. Barefoot is, simply put, an extraordinary individual." Philip Sharples, President Sharples Industries Inc. Tubac, Arizona.

"I have known Bob Barefoot for three years during which time he has provided my spouse with critical information. As a result of this relationship, I was able to introduce dozens of people to Mr. Barefoot's idea relative to critical illness and nutrition. The results achieved have been remarkable. It is my personal opinion that Mr. Barefoot is the absolute top of his field, nutritional therapy." W. Grant Fairley, The Fairley Erker Group, Edmonton, Canada.

"I am a chemist and have been involved in product development, specifically nutritional supplements. I have written numerous articles and lectured throughout the United States on these products and the benefits of utilizing alternative medicine and alternative medical products within the U.S. healthcare regimen. Over the past three years I have traveled and lectured with Mr. Barefoot on numerous occasions all over the United States. He is recognized as a world class expert on calcium and its nutritional benefits for the human body. Mr. Barefoot blends his prestige and uncanny ability to talk to the average person in a way that allows complicated scientific subjects to be completely understandable and accepted. I have seen Mr. Barefoot's information help a lot of people." Alex Nobles, Executive Vice President, Benchmark USA Inc., Salt Lake.

11

"I have been associated with Mr. Barefoot since 1993. His nutrition therapy is the result of twenty years of research into non-invasive treatment of generic diseases. In Canada we now have six M.D.'s practicing his protocols. I understand that numerous Russian M.D.'s in Moscow are also practicing his protocols. This number will increase exponentially as the testimonial success of hundreds of afflicted people becomes known. Mr. Barefoot's biochemistry and science brings credence to his recommended dietary and lifestyle protocols. He must be considered at the top of his field," Peter Epp. P. Eng., President Albritco Development Corporation, Calgary, Canada.

"I am the General Manager of an audio cassette tape manufacturer. Previously, I was the Vice President of an engineering consulting company specializing in nuclear technology analysis under contract to the U.S. government. With a BS degree in Electrical Engineering, graduate school work at UCLA and over 10 years of research at McDonnell Douglas, my technical and scientific tools are extensive. I currently specialize in the audio production of technical information specializing in nutrition and health. It is in this regard that I have come to know the reputation and work of Robert Barefoot. Our company actively seeks men and women with scientific and medical backgrounds in order to develop substantive resource material for our client base. Robert Barefoot's lectures, books and tapes support his position as a leading spokesperson for the benefits of nutrition for good health." Al Vendetti, General Manager, Exxel Audio Productions, Oceanside, California.

"I am the founder of a company that specializes in both mining and the export of health and nutritional products overseas. Mr. Barefoot has tremendous knowledge of

biochemistry and his expertise in the field of calcium research has earned him recognition worldwide for both his lecturing and his research. He has authored several books, which my company exports overseas as nutritional standards for people involved in the nutrition industry. He has also researched and developed calcium supplements, which are being exported to several countries abroad. His research of the relationship between disease and nutrition is gaining recognition worldwide and if properly implemented, could substantially reduce the devastating effects of degenerative diseases caused by mineral and vitamin deficiency." Brett R. Davies, President, Davies International, Denver, Colorado.

"I am well known in the area of nutrition. I am certified by the National Association of Health Care Professionals as a Health Care Councilor and have lectured extensively in the United States, Canada, Russia and the Ukraine. Mr. Barefoot is considered one of the most knowledgeable people in the world, on effects of calcium on health." Robert G. Bremner, Mechanicsville, Virginia.

"Mr. Barefoot is a man in pursuit of "Excellence," in all his endeavors. He has received wide recognition for his research in the biochemistry field, dealing with malnutrition. I have the distinct privilege and pleasure of having known Mr. Barefoot for several years," Jerry R. Gallion, International Financier, Vaulx Milieu, France.

"I am a retired university professor, Ph.D., known in the field of Pharmaceutical Chemistry, having written and lectured extensively over a forty year period, publishing numerous scientific articles. Based on Mr. Barefoot's education, and background in chemistry and nutrition, along

13

with his published books and lecturing, it is my professional opinion that Mr. Barefoot is near the top of his field." Jerry Rollins, Ph.D., Austin, Texas.

"We have purchased two of your books, "The Calcium Factor" and "Death By Diet." INCREDIBLE BOOKS! Well worth reading by EVERY PERSON IN AMERICA OF READING AGE !! I HAVE READ THEM TWICE.

We totally discount the crap that the "fanatics" in other fields and in the government who discount your writings. It <u>does show how afraid they are of the TRUTH, doesn't it</u> ? Bob we feel that your sales of coral calcium have helped so many people (including ourselves) and should continue unabated. Our congratulations to you for writing the EXCELLENT information you have in those books, and, therefore, helping to benefit many, many, many people's health.

We wish unabated success for you continuing your writings, work and success in defeating the scared idiots." Mae and Al Schone, Felton PA.

"After seeing you being interviewed on television and hearing your story about coral calcium, I bought your books and a supply of coral calcium. I read the books with much interest. I have taken vitamin and mineral supplements for years and have read a number of books to learn more about vitamins, etc. In the 70's I was able to rid myself of bone spurs in my neck by increasing my calcium intake, just like you said in your books, after a friend told me that it was a lack of calcium that caused bone spurs. However, it took me three years to do it. Your books woke me up to the fact that our body does not absorb nearly enough calcium, and most of us never give it a chance to do so. The amounts that I was taking were "recommended" levels and in spite of the supplements, I have

arthritis in my knee and bone spurs in my shoulder, and I have sinusitis and a long list of allergies.

After only three weeks on coral calcium I have eliminated 99% of the pain associated with an arthritic left knee and a right shoulder with bone spurs. I walk naturally again, and for the past year I had required a cane to walk. The only thing that I have done differently since reading your books is switch to coral calcium. My energy level is much higher. I look forward to seeing my health improve even further. Thank you so much for getting the word out on coral calcium and giving us a chance to help us cure ourselves. The chemistry involved, explained in layman's terms in your books, showed me just how vital calcium is and encourages me to stay on the regimen." Kennith R. Davis, Nashville, TN

Foreword

By Scott Miller
The Mineral Man

During a career which oft times has cast me into the quixotic world of holistic, natural, organic, and herbal remedies and supplements, I have encountered a vast array of individuals who profess to have control over, or possession of, or exclusive access to... THE SOLUTION to mankind's mental and physical maladies. With rare exceptions, the passion and zeal with which these individuals promote their particular product(s) are derived from the most basic economic stimulus; profit in pursuit of riches.

Not the case with Bob Barefoot, which is why I am both flattered and gratified that he asked me to write this forward. Although Bob is a passionate zealot in the promotion of his beliefs, he is a singular rarity in my personal experience in that his best interests economically are constantly sacrificed in support of his cause; which may be defined simply as the promotion of coral calcium as a significant source of longevity and health. In fact, were coral calcium not the subject matter, it would be easy to substitute a religious context and cast Bob in the light of itinerate preacher for Bob is constantly "on the stump." He travels tirelessly throughout North America, often at his own expense, preaching his "gospel" of coral calcium supplementation. He rarely accepts honoraria, asking only travel, food and lodging costs. To be sure he has income from other business interests, but he is far from a rich man in monetary terms. But he is rich nonetheless in that he has identified that most precious human commodity; he has found his passion in life ... and for over 30 years he has continued to pursue it, nurture it and live it with relentless, all consuming, single minded fervor.

Having said that, however, my assignation as regards this book requires that my admiration for Bob Barefoot, the man be separate from my support of his conclusions as a scientist. Bob is a chemist who has published several scientific articles on analytical chemistry and mineral diagenesis. In addition he has developed and patented several methods of biochemical hydrocarbon extraction for the petroleum industry and metal extraction for the mining industry. As he will explain, his application of biochemical research in these fields, although seemingly unrelated at the time, led him to investigate the relationship between disease and nutrition. This work led him to publish *The Calcium Factor* and *Death By Diet* books, which identified mineral intake as a crucial factor in health maintenance and longevity.

In this book Bob offers a cohesive scientific argument that specific nutritional deficiency is the cause of cancer, diabetes and heart disease (the Big Three) among many others, and offers a compelling argument that correcting these deficiencies can result in both prevention and reversal. From there we are led to the specific composite structure of coral calcium harvested from the waters surrounding the Ryukyu Islands in Okinawa and the conclusion that this specific natural storehouse of vital micronutrients may well hold the key to the well-being of mankind.

17

Heavy stuff to be sure, and while Bob presents a detailed account of his concepts and findings, he is the first to admit the current limitations of the body of knowledge that exists to explain the biological actions of this marvel of marine medicine. At the same time there exists substantial evidence throughout Europe for the successful therapeutic use of a variety of corals from this region that stretch back over several centuries. Add to that Japanese reports comprised of 600 years of scientific and folklore literature in such voluminous content that it cannot be ignored. Further to that one must acknowledge conclusive American studies that acknowledge the importance of calcium in particular and minerals in general for health and disease prevention.

Finally, let it be said that Bob has committed to more than 30 years of his life to the nutritional application of calcium and minerals. His passion not withstanding he has, by any standard, approached this discussion of coral calcium with objective science. He has studied the chemical composition of every known commercially accessible coral deposit. He has investigated extensively the anti-cancer and anti-microbial properties reported with the use of coral. He is a man of science and discipline by education and training. His professional reputation is at risk with every book or theory or hypothesis he presents. Above all his economic well-being is not dependent on the sale of this book or the sale of coral calcium. His singular goal is the attainment of wellness for mankind.

It is with these facts in that I implore you, the reader, whether layperson of professional, to enjoy this book in health; carefully ponder its content in the light of several hundred years of documented history and take action as it suggests. To do so will have a positive impact on you and your loved ones' health and well-being.

— G Scott Miller, Arizona, 2001

G. Scott Miller is a semi-retired executive living in Arizona who is known most prominently in health and nutrition circles as "The Mineral Man." His contributions in that arena include the development of America's largest selling liquid mineral dietary supplement.

Preface

For over two decades, Bob Barefoot has been known as a *medical maverick*, because of his choice to both live and research preventive medicine. He is not a stranger to controversy and debate. Having started his career in pure chemistry and related sciences, he became fascinated by the bigger picture on how physical science can explain many aspects of the complexities of biological systems. The turning point in his career was his interaction with the late Dr. Carl Reich M.D., first as a scientist and subsequently as a collaborative researcher. The wisdom of Dr. Carl Reich's observations on the importance of calcium for health attracted much debate. In fact his revolutionary proposals on the role of calcium as a versatile and potent bio-element that can prevent and treat many diseases were so challenging to his peers that he suffered oppression, rejection and ridicule while his patients were experiencing almost miraculous cures. Then, in 1984 Dr. Carl Reich lost his license for claiming that calcium supplements cure cancer, a claim that is echoed by many of our best medical researchers today. Just prior to his death, City Scope magazine in Calgary did a feature article entitled *"Ahead of His Time,"* in which they credit Dr. Reich with the passage of Bill #209, the Province of Alberta Medical Profession Amendment Act, which states that *"a practitioner shall not be found guilty of unbecoming conduct or found to be incapable or unfit to practice medicine solely on the basis that the practitioner employs a therapy that is non-traditional or departs from the prevailing medical practices, unless it can be demonstrated by medical authorities that the therapy has a*

20

safety risk for that patient unreasonably greater than the prevailing treatment."

The History of medicine is replete with examples of the hazards that scientists face when they propose a theory that may not be palatable to prevailing bodies of opinion. Dr. Reich showed, by a lifetime of practical treatment experience, that calcium and other minerals play a vital role in the biology of life. Whilst we would like to believe that modern science is more open to *"new"* suggestions or *"reactivated interest"* in rejected theories, the modern day questioning of prevailing bodies of medical opinion seems to be equally as hazardous for many researchers as it was several centuries ago.

The phenomenon of the *"lone hero against the world"* is sometimes used as an excuse to gain unjustified support for alternative scientific thoughts, but powerful economic influences act against the obvious introduction of simple natural options for health maintenance. Healthcare in the West is dominated by allopathic (conventional) thinking which tends to focus on pharmaceutical developments and classical surgical strategies. The incentives to engage in preventive medicine are not as powerful as those to treat established disease with proprietary technology that generates staggering profits. Fortunately modern medicine is changing as more individuals demand alternatives. Some conventional approaches to disease prevention or treatment may on occasion result in dubious success.

The title of this book *Barefoot on Coral Calcium* tells a story. Barefoot stands on coral calcium as a unique and valuable marine miracle for health as well as, in his opinion, the best calcium supplement available. Whilst the act of standing on stony coral may be painful, the value of this positioning for health promotion is worth the discomfort! Coral calcium is a *"powerhouse of health"* giving mineral nutrients that combine to support all body chemistry. The value of abundant nutrient minerals for disease prevention and longevity has been well described in both folklore and scientific literature. Coral calcium has over 600 years of history with millions of people who took or are currently taking the nutrient, including thousands and thousands of testimonials about its health benefits. Whilst calcium is a key constituent of coral calcium, coral calcium is a source of several other essential mineral nutrients including substantial amounts of magnesium, zinc, strontium, boron and many more.

My book on coral calcium is the culmination of three decades of research. There are several communities throughout the world who enjoy health and longevity to a greater degree than humankind. The common denominator in this phenomenon is not their sedentary lifestyle and the fact that they eat fish, fruits and vegetables, as those cultures that live nearby and do the same do not have the same health benefits, but rather it is the abundant mineral supply in their diet, especially calcium. The inhabitants of Okinawa in Japan are one example of this status of *"super health and well-being,"* Japanese scientists have concluded that the good health and longevity of the people of Okinawa is due to their consumption of calcium-rich coral water, and the Spanish Explorers filled their ship holds with coral calcium that they concluded was the source of the good health.

In an article in the January 1973 edition of *National Geographic* entitled, **"Search For The Oldest People"** provided examples of many of these cultures including the Abkhasians from Georgia (high in the mountains), the Hunzas of Pakistan (high in the mountains), and the Vilcabambans of Ecuador (high in the mountains). This list was quickly expanded to include the Bamas in China (high in the mountains), the Azerbaijans (high in the mountains), the Armenians (high in the mountains), the Tibetans (high in the mountains), and the Titicacas of Peru (high in the mountains). To this list, of couse the Okinawans of Japan (sea level) must be added.

With all of the above cultures, *disease virtually does not exist:* "almost" no cancer, no heart disease, no diabetes, no Alzheimer's, no arthritis, etc. For example the Okinawans have less than one fifth the heart disease that Americans do. These cultures have no mental disorders and no doctors. They also live much longer than we do in North America and their aging process is dramatically slower. For example the Okinawans live 8 years longer than mainland Japan who lives 4 years longer than Americans. And the elderly seem to have youthful bodies. The common denominator is that all of their water is loaded with mineral nutrients from melting glaciers high in the mountains, and from the disintegrating coral reefs in Okinawa. One quart of Hunza water, in Pakistan, contains 17,000 milligrams of calcium (17 times the RDA at the time), which is also equivalent to 17 quarts of milk, and they drink several quarts each day. In general, the over riding factor in their disease-free longevity is the fact that these cultures can consume almost *"one hundred times the RDA"* of everything, with the only side effect being great health and longevity. Also, they eat large amounts of everything we are told is not good for you such as butter, salt, eggs, milk and animal fat.

Another major factor is that these cancer-free people are in the sun, which we are told causes cancer. While Black Africans spend most of every day naked in the sun and are almost cancer-free, Black Americans, who avoid the sun like the plague, are ravished by cancer and are almost at double the risk of cancer as are White Americans who sunbathe. Mr. Barefoot and Dr. Carl Reich wrote the book, *The Calcium Factor* which detailed the scientific explanations for this cancer phenomenon and for the remarkable health and youth of others. The book was published in 1992. Mr. Barefoot was immediately invited as a guest speaker at health shows and was a frequent guest on numerous radio and television talk shows. Ten years later, in 2002, he was to make two of the most watched infomercials in television history, making a dramatic impact on nutrition in America.

I am hoping that when you read this book, you will discover the reasoning behind minerals for good health. I found the Japanese to be warm and kind people with great integrity and they are willing to share with the world their marine miracle, coral calcium. In Japanese folklore, for hundreds of years, they have taught that the islands of Okinawa will one day *"cure the world."*

— Robert R. Barefoot, Wickenburg, Arizona, 2001

Acknowledgement

The author is grateful and wishes to acknowledge his appreciation for the dedication, contributions and efforts of Fay Harlin, Barney Woods, John Baker his best friend and wife Isabelle, Bruce and Carole Downey, and most of all, his cherished wife of 35 years, Karen Barefoot, in assisting the completion, critical review and editing of this publication.

Notation

Although this publication is intended to direct the attention of both the physician and the patient to the torrent of scientific research being carried out on the significance of biological calcium, it is not the intention of the authors to provide an alternative to the orthodox physician-patient relationship. Rather, it is the objective of the authors to expand the dimensions of orthodox medicine itself, and help speed it towards medical practices of the twenty-first century where diet and lifestyle will play a predominant role in preventive medicine.

"If the doctors of today do not become the dieticians of tomorrow, the dieticians of today will become the doctors of tomorrow." (Rockefeller Institute of Medical Research).

Post Script

Because so many people who are suffering and in pain have sought my help, I have become passionate about ending degenerative disease. I have seen the success of using God's nutrients and I know that the results can be explained in detail in scientific terms. Both God and Science are One. However, if we start to cure disease we should start with those most affected, the Black community in America. Because of my passion, many in the Black community have tried to get Oprah Winfrey to talk to me, but unfortunately, she has a wall of protection around her that decides for her what she should hear. If she would one day be able to listen, my message for her would be, "Let's cure humanity, starting with Black America first."

I also would like to challenge each and every celebrity in America to look, listen and learn, and then to do what is right as America will eagerly follow you. Thus, you have the ability to end suffering and misery in America. All you have to do is to try God's nutrients after you read this book. You will discover the magic and when you tell your fellow Americans, they will gladly listen and follow your example. The result will be a disease-free America. You owe it to your country to try.

CHAPTER 1

Coral Minerals and Health

In Search of Health and Youth

I share everyone's quest for health and longevity. Whilst humankind has been denied a simple *"fountain of youth,"* modern science is pointing us towards the possibility of using nutrition to help secure a long and healthy life. In this new millennium, the limitations of allopathic (conventional) medicine have become increasingly apparent.

The proverbial quest for the *"fountain of youth"* did not begin with the Spanish explorer, Ponce de Leon, but it is more than a coincidence that coral calcium was introduced as a important treatment agent in the oldest pharmacy Europe that is located in Spain. This pharmacy is now a museum in Penaranda de Duero in Northern Spain and it was established in 1685. The introduction of ground coral as one of the first pharmaceuticals in Spain may have occurred from earlier occupation of the Iberian Peninsula by the Moors (Arabs). In this Medieval Pharmacy ground, stony coral is *prominently displayed* as a treatment. The dispensing container of coral bears several inscriptions that describe its beneficial effects on the heart and brain.

The use of coral in early forms of allopathic (conventional) medicine was based on little more than empiric (trial and error) use with evidence of benefit. When the Spanish found the inhabitants of Okinawa to be unusually healthy and long living, they recognized that the ingestion of coral sand, later to be renamed coral calcium, was the prime ingredient. In contemporary medicine, we still operate by trial and error, but we are convinced that we can better measure outcomes using modern scientific principles of research. Whilst I do not doubt the ability of modern science to identify the safety and effectiveness of modern medicines, the precedence of the successful use of coral calcium for health speaks for itself.

It is foolish to propose that any single agent will promote health and longevity in a consistent and simple manner. After all, aging and disease development are highly complex biological events with a multitude of contributory factors. However, it should be noted that coral cannot be considered a *"single agent,"* as it is composed of thousands of different skeletal organisms that leached nutrients out of the ocean for millions of years, thereby containing all of the mineral nutrients contained in the human body. Setting these technical thoughts aside, humankind has been on a perpetual search for one potion, lotion or elixir that will guarantee eternal youth. Whilst this miracle eludes discovery, some of the secrets of health and longevity may be much more simple than hitherto supposed.

Lifestyle and Minerals

Implicit in the desire for eternal youth is our wish to avoid poor health which seems to emerge with advancing age. Of all interventions that have been tried for enhancing well-being and long-life, few have worked. I believe that the

28

issues are tied up in our lifestyle. The biblical patriarchs, who definitely had a different lifestyle, lived to be over 900 years old. Today, a healthy lifestyle is a key factor in extended life that must have a quality free from disease. Beyond the important, health sermons on cigarette smoking, stress, drug abuse etc., nutritional factors figure most strongly as determinants of health and well-being. The avoidance of all adverse lifestyle is advisable, but the domain of lifestyle most amenable to correction is *"sound and appropriate nutrition."*

It is easy for a chemist (like myself) to see the body as a <u>universe</u> of interacting chemicals. Whilst this perception provides an incomplete picture of life, it is a good start to understanding the importance of minerals as a vital component of a diet for health, as each mineral must serve at least one specific biological function. With the exception of aluminum and silicon, the human body is made up of the same minerals, <u>including gold,</u> in differing amounts as the Earth. I shall present evidence that mineral balance (especially calcium) in the body is an absolute prerequisite for health and longevity, but I trust this important advice will not be taken in isolation of instructions on a healthy lifestyle.

Why Coral Minerals?

In my earlier writings, I have stressed the calcium factor for health and many of these issues will be further addressed in later chapters of this book. My belief in the role of coral minerals for health has come from many years of careful research and observation of its effects in thousands of individuals who have used coral products. There is a voluminous amount of folklore, historical and scientific literature on stony corals and their biological implications, but I have been most impressed by its apparent *universal health benefits* which on occasion, <u>almost</u> defy explanation. My support for the nutraceutical value of coral calcium is not a *"leap of faith"* based on my channeled research on calcium alone. When coral calcium from Okinawa and surrounding domains in Japan is used as a food supplement, it touches many lives in a highly positive manner (Chapter 9).

In brief, we can learn from the experiences of the inhabitants of Okinawa who have among the best health and longest lives in the world, which include ten times as many centenarians as areas found in the United States. (see Chapter 3) and large numbers of robust individuals in their eighties and nineties. Whilst many factors may operate to create this desirable circumstance, I, like the Spanish explorers before me, believe a key to this circumstance is the use of coral calcium as a food supplement in this highly blessed community of people. Whilst some people may dismiss this phenomenon as a chance observation, there are new scientific and medical discoveries that give a credible, scientific basis for the use of coral calcium for health. One key constituent of coral calcium is readily absorbable calcium and magnesium, but other factors within coral, including its highly balanced mineral content and the occurrence of microbes, may account for observed benefits. Beyond these issues are speculations about other components of coral and a clear recognition that <u>many of the</u> minerals are present in a *"chemical form"* that is highly desirable for use by the body – vide infra (refer to the following).

Returning to "The Calcium Factor"

In my earlier book entitled *The Calcium Factor,* I present viewpoints <u>and statistics</u> that may not be wholeheartedly embraced by conventional medicine. My clear focus in my earlier book was to highlight the underestimated importance of calcium for health. No healer would doubt the essential nature of calcium, which is the most abundant mineral in the human body, for health, especially related to its role in signaling biochemical processes in cells, controlling muscle contractions, initiating DNA synthesis, and building bones. However, the general level of calcium intake in the Western diet is much lower in many people than is required for optimal health. Furthermore, there are many other ancillary actions of calcium, such as the critical control of the pH (acidity or alkalinity) of the body fluids. This is demonstrated by the fact that body fluids become more acidic with aging when calcium is lacking in the diet. This results in the expulsion of oxygen which can lead to numerous diseases, such as cancer, according to two-time Nobel Prize winner Otto Warburg.

I have referred to calcium as the **"King of the Bioelements,"** where deficiency of this element is invariably associated with a whole host of diseases. Calcium, however, does not act alone in the body. It has to be present in abundance with other minerals and cofactors (especially magnesium and vitamin D), in order that it can play its pivotal role in health. The *"secrets"* of coral calcium for health become unwrapped as we begin to explore the role of coral minerals in supporting the chemistry of life.

Clues on Longevity, Health and Minerals

My personal odyssey to define the link between minerals and health was reinforced by knowledge that certain geographical locations in the world had inhabitants who were strangers to illness and lived to a ripe, old age. Among these longevous people are Abkasians from Georgia, the

Hunzas of Pakistan, the Bamas of China, the Vilcabambans of Ecuador and certain Azerbaijans. These small populations seem to share a common factor that they live at high altitude. Living at high elevation presents an ecology where melting glacial water has an abundant mineral content, for example each quart of Hunza water contains about 20,000 milligrams of calcium, and these people drink several quarts each day. I believe that the common denominator in this group is that their diet is high in mineral nutrients that are derived from melting glaciers and snow. Many other scientists, such as Dr. Joe Wallach, have proposed this mineral factor in longevity.

This association between abundant mineral intake and health is supported by the finding that sea level populations with health and longevity, such as the Okinawans in Japan, have a similar abundance of minerals in their diet. In the case of Okinawans the source is the offerings of the coral reefs around the Ryukyu islands. These reefs provide mineral enrichment to the water supply and coral is often taken as a supplement in the diet. Again, one could claim an "interesting" coincidence, but after a while the many coincidences start to imply proof of cause and effect.

Whilst minerals may not be the whole story of health and longevity. I believe that they are much more important than has been previously supposed. There has been a tendency in modern medicine to reject remedies of natural origin, such as coral, that have centuries of precedence of successful use. The pendulum is now swinging in the opposite direction as pluralistic medicine emerges and we move back to basics in applying optimum lifestyle and nutrition for health. Coral calcium serves as an historical example of a natural agent from the ancient seas which holds great power for health and well-being.

CHAPTER 2

The Bio-Synthesis of the Seas

Life in Water

Scientists may have tended to underestimate the importance of the oceans in sustaining life on our planet. The complex and varied composition of the oceans of the world make them home to more living organisms than the land. Water forms an ideal medium to contain all of the inorganic and organic materials that are essential for the development and sustenance of life forms. The *"vitality factors"* contained within oceans, rivers and land-locked collections of water are the most important component of the food chain of all plant and animal life. The healing properties of sea water have been recognized by every culture for thousands of years. In some circumstances *"treated sea water"* has been used as medicine with variable benefit. In wartime, it was successfully used in lieu of blood for transfusions.

About 80% (four-fifths) of the total animal life on the planet exists in the seas. Plant life is also abundant and seaweeds (especially kelp) are among the fastest growing most prolific plants on earth. The biomasses vary in density throughout the ocean. The deepest parts of the ocean supports life forms about which we know very little. The concept of *"biomass"* is important in oceanographic studies and it refers to the amount of living matter found per unit area of the sea. Underwater sea forests of kelp and coral reefs are rich biomasses that support a high concentration of living organisms. Coral reefs grow over thousands of years and mature into a rich ecology where nutrients and elements are concentrated. If the oceans are considered a soup of life, the underwater forests, the coral reefs and the seabeds are the dumplings in the soup. These *"dumplings"* are huge *"vitalistic"* aggregations.

Whilst we are still exploring the landmass of the earth, the oceans hold many secrets that are relatively inaccessible. This under-explored frontier of waters of the world's surface has a volume of 42 million billion cubic ft or 286 million cubic miles. Experts believe, for instance, that the average gold content is 0.012 parts per billion. This calculates out to be 460,000,000,000 ounces of gold or over 100 times the gold currently held in the world's vaults. Thus, the oceans are an enormous collection of metals, minerals and chemical substances that sustain life. The seas contain many factors that are produced by its own living organisms.

An analysis of sea water shows variable results depending on the site of collection. However, it contains a striking array of organic compounds derived from plant and animal life. These compounds include organic acids, sterols, carotenoids, various free enzymes and variable amounts of macro and micronutrients (fats, carbohydrates and proteins). Aggregations of life forms in the oceans, such as coral reefs, concentrate these complex compounds. It is easy to appreciate that the coral reefs are composed of, or exposed to, all nutrient classes known to man.

The sea is rich in salt (sodium chloride) and every

natural element known to man is present at one or other location. The contents of the sea are determined to a major degree by its residents, but oceans have many citizens who live in different geographic locations with distinct climates. Thus, diverse ecology in the seas mirrors the diversity of life that is encountered on landmasses of the earth.

Reciprocal Harmony of Life in the Seas

The sea contains a massive expanse of life, which it supports by its content of *"free -floating"* minerals and bio-active, nutritional compounds. Water provides an ideal communication pathway for messenger molecules of life. There are free floating hormones in some areas of the sea that are elaborated by certain marine organisms. These *ecto-hormones* (ecto means "from outside") can be taken up by various other plants or life-forms in the ocean and cause many biological chain reactions that support the diverse array of marine inhabitants.

The chemical balance in the oceans supports life in complex ways. Therefore, one cannot be surprised by scientific reports that many marine life forms and their environmental waters or habitants, such as coral reefs, produce substances that have potent and versatile biological actions in nature. Marine compounds of various types have been found to be antifungal, antibiotic, anticancer, antiviral, growth inhibiting, analgesic, cardio-stimulatory (or inhibitory) and antiangiogenic in their actions.

To add to our appreciation of the health secrets that the oceans contain is the recognition that four-fifths of all life on our planet (about one-half million species) lives in water. Massive amounts of suspended organic matter are incorporated into the food chain of marine organisms. Furthermore, marine organisms, such as living corals or mussels, process or expose their life cycle to thousands of tons of water. In one estimate, a small colony of mussels (ten million) can process one square mile of seawater that is 25' deep. As *"big fish eats little fish"* or marine organisms are used in complex food chains, the permutations of transfer of active molecules becomes limitless. Humankind joins this complex harmony of planetary life when it harvests the offerings of the oceans.

Origins of Life in Water

The depths of the oceans present a daunting task for explorers. With advances in engineering, submersible vehicles (submarines) have allowed exploration of the depths of the oceans. Much pioneering work with remotely operated vehicles (ROVs) has allowed exploration of the abyssal planes of the oceans. As diverse as the marine life is, the variation of *"climatic"* conditions in the oceans is vast. The life in the oceans is very different at different depths of water. Whilst warm oceans, closer to sunlight have abundant plant and other marine life, the depths of the oceans have been found to be teeming with primitive life forms.

Explorations of underwater topography such has volcanoes beneath the oceans have given some clues about the origin of life itself. In several distinct areas of the ocean, there are deep-sea vents that emit mineral enriched, hot water from interactions with earth's core. These vents provide *"chemical energy"* rather than *"light energy"* to support life. Most life on earth is supported by light energy which drives photosynthesis.

Bacteria and primitive life forms that thrive in and around these underwater vents have basic *"genetic material"* that suggests that they are related to all organisms on the earth. In other words, the genetic material or nucleic acid (RNA) found in these organisms is similar to that in all animal life. This finding has led to new proposals about the origin of life on earth. It has been proposed that life developed in warm sea waters, perhaps around these submersed vents. Life is believed to have begun in the seas about 3.3 billion years ago and studies of deep sea communities regularly *"turn up"* new species of organisms.

Drugs and Dietary Supplements from the Sea

Many drugs and nutrients have been derived from marine sources, but the health secrets of the oceans remain sadly underexplored. For examples, marine sources of omega 3 fatty acids are essential nutrients that have wide ranging health benefits including the promotion of cardiovascular health, immune function and optimal structure and function of the central nervous system. Extracts of coral have been shown to have antibacterial and anti-inflammatory properties, in addition to the value of coral calcium as a mineral source. Table 1 gives examples of biopharmaceuticals from the sea.

Table 1
Examples of Biopharmaceuticals from Marine Sources

CLASS OF PHARMACEUTICAL	EXAMPLES
Minerals/Vitamins	Coral calcium, oyster shells, cod liver oil, shark oils, kelp, seaweeds, etc.

Antibiotics	Crassin and Eunic from corals. Ectyonin from Sponges. Cephalosporins from fungi.
Antiinflammatory agents	Erythrolides A and B from soft coral. Pseudopteractans A-C from soft coral.
Antihelminthic agents	Domoic acid, kainic acid from red algae.
Antibacterial/antiviral compounds	Paolin I and II from oysters, clams and squid. Anti-ulcer/anti-peptic agents. Carageenan and agar.
Anticancer agents	Discodermalide from deep water sponges. Extracts of shark cartilage and shark liver oil (alkylglycerols). Insecticides. Nereistoxin from sea worms.

Structure of Corals

Corals belong to the phylum (group) of marine organisms called Cnidaria (Coelenterata) which also includes jellyfish, sea anemones and hydroids. These organisms tend to be symmetrical with a digestive tract that has one single opening. They possess a *"nematocyst"* or stinging apparatus which contains and protects the coral polyp with venom of varying potency. The stony corals are named because they secrete a supporting exoskeleton (outside hard structure). This stony covering contains the soft structures of the living coral polyps. These living corals form reefs which support a large biomass. In tropical waters and some temperate zones these corals proliferate to a vast degree that builds islands. A classic example of this geographic phenomenon is the infrastructure of the island chains in and around Okinawa, Japan.

Coral calcium is derived from reef-building coral and it is harvested from the pristine waters off the Nansei Islands (Rukuyuku and Satsunan), Japan. These islands spread towards the southeast from the southern tip of Japan's main land mass towards Taiwan. Using careful, harvesting techniques that are sustaining for the environment, several companies collect and process coral calcium for use as a food supplement. The Japanese government supervises this collection process and they provide special certification to certain types of coral. Under a microscope, coral appears as tubes, horns and honeycombs. It has the appearance of an abandoned city. Coral calcium has been officially recognized by the Japanese government as a valuable food supplement. This official standing was registered by Japan in July 1989, but the coral sands have enjoyed thousands of years of local use as an important source of health giving nutrients in the diet of Okinawans. It was discovered by the early Spanish explorers, 500 years ago, who filled their ship holds with the coral sands. The chemists in Spain, attempting to discover the reason for its miraculous curative properties, discovered that the main ingredient was calcium, so they renamed it *"coral calcium."* Today, tens of millions of people around the world consume coral calcium daily.

Different Types of Coral Calcium

It is important to recognize that two broad, but distinct types of coral calcium, are used as health giving supplements by the Japanese and many people throughout the world. The first type is fossilized calcium that has been deposited on the land mass, or washed up on to beaches. The second type is taken directly from the seabed. The seabed coral is the coral that has dropped from the reef or is processed by reef inhabitants. This type of *"coral sand"* has been washed to the ocean floor by wave actions. Marine coral is closer in composition to the living forms of corals, because the marine microbes are still active and many minerals and organic elements are retained, in comparison to fossilized, land-based coral.

There are important differences in composition between fossilized (land-based) coral and marine (seabed) coral. Marine coral contains more magnesium, and the balance of calcium (24%) to magnesium (12%) content of this second type of marine coral is close to 2:1. This 2 to 1 ratio is the ideal ratio for calcium and magnesium intake in the human diet. My research has led me to believe strongly that the natural, magnesium enriched, marine coral is to be strongly preferred as a health giving supplement over land based (fossilized coral), which contains less than 1% magnesium. This superiority is due to its retained, ideal, ionic balance of calcium and magnesium in a 2:1 ratio, and the fact that a host of other nutrients were also washed out during weathering processes. These issues are considered in greater detail in Chapter 4.

Linking "Life-Supporting" Concepts and Coral

To understand the potential of coral for health, one needs to understand the ecology of life on coral collections in the ocean. Coral reefs have been dated back over two hundred million years and they are the largest structures on Earth created by any living organism. The beauty of coral reefs hide a secret that up to one half of all species of fish in the ocean live or visit the biomass around coral. In addition to fish, the coral reef contains hundreds of thousands of different species of bacteria, fungi, invertebrate organisms and plants, which interact in a harmonious manner.

What is the Structure of a Coral Reef?

Coral reefs are sea mountains of minerals of which calcium carbonate predominates, along with numerous other inorganic and organic forms of calcium. Calcium is a biological glue and an inorganic building block that is ubiquitous on the planet earth. In order to build a reef, the living coral polyps require specific climatic and ecologic conditions. Indeed, coral reefs are most preponderant in warm waters of the ocean which have a range of temperature from 20°C to 30°C, approximately. Without sunlight the living infrastructure of organisms on the reef that use photo-synthesis for nutrition cannot survive. These photosynthetic organisms (zooanthellae–algae) are quite primitive, but efficient in forming a basic nutrient source for the food chain of the reef dwellers. Some marine organisms rely heavily on the photosynthesizing organisms. For example, coral reef sponges obtain the bulk of their nutrients from these organisms and some species of jellyfish harbor photosynthesizers in their tentacles.

Of the vast number of species of coral, two distinct, basic types are recognized. These are the reef-building stony corals and the more delicate soft corals that have an inner skeleton. Not all corals from aggregations into colonies and many soft corals live among the stony corals. The most interesting aspect of coral is their efficient and versatile ability to reproduce. They can reproduce by budding in an asexual manner and many polyps can form with remaining connections to its forerunner. Once a year, the corals may spawn filling areas of the reef with *massive amounts of eggs and sperm* (the reefs are submerged in a cloud of sperm and eggs) which attract plankton-eating fish and mammals.

Oceanographers refer to several distinct types of coral reef. The coral reefs in Okinawa are associated with dormant underwater volcanoes and they tend to grow outwards to maintain their submersion in the seas. Fringing reefs are raised from coastal plain seabeds and can be found in the Caribbean and the Great Barrier Reef. Reefs can grow with amazing variations in architecture that is shaped by the geological circumstances and climate of the ocean.

Life on the Reef

The miraculous chains of life events on coral reefs is highly complex. The basic photosynthetic organisms and plant life provide food for herbivorous (vegetarian) inhabitants such as damsel fish, parrotfish, blennies and puffer fish. The parrotfish play a unique role in the biomass of reefs. They use their strong teeth to chew away at coral which is ground in their digestive tract and released to form the grand-up, sandy bases of the reef. In fact, parrotfish and similar *"coral munchers"* are a prime source of marine coral that is harvested as coral calcium. The reef has many species that sleep by night and play by day or vice versa. The coral reef has a fascinating bio-rhythm with an interplay of thousands of species of fish, worms, sponges, fungi and transient visitors. The recognition of the diversity of life and dynamic life forces to which coral is exposed makes it easier to understand how difficult it may be to define all of the nutrient benefits that may come from coral. There is much that we do not know about the dynamics of life surrounding coral.

Chapter Summary

Before we explore the chemical composition of coral and its nutritional content, its origin and complexities of development must be appreciated. Coral polyps are clever builders of underwater domains that are teaming with plant and animal life. Of major interest is the observation of longevity and health of the inhabitants of the reef islands of Okinawa, Japan. These islands are a source of coral calcium that has a long recorded history of use as a health-giving food supplement.

CHAPTER 3

The Elixir(s) of Life in Okinawa (Japan)

Longevity in Okinawa

Okinawa, composed of hundreds of coral reef islands, is located at the southern tip of the mainland of Japan. It is a Prefecture (Province) with approximately one and one-half million inhabitants. Native Okinawans are among the most healthy and longest living people in the world. Recent population statistics show that Okinawa has more centenarians than other parts of Japan, and ten times as many per capita as the United States. Japan itself is noted for longevity, but Okinawa stands out as a special location for health, well-being and *elite elderly* inhabitants. The average number of people at or over the age of 100 years is 28.86 per 100.000 of the population compared with the national, Japanese average of 8.92 per 100.000 people. This compares with about 3 per 100,000 of the population in the United States. In the late 1990's approximately 400 people in Okinawa were recorded to be living beyond their 100th birthday, and those in their 80's and 90's lead extremely robust, active, healthy, and productive lives. This longevity among Okinawans is striking.

More Legends of Okinawa

It is recorded in folklore and legends that an Emperor

of China sent a mission of three thousand explorers to find the land of *"heaven on earth."* This heavenly place was called *"Horai"* — according to legend – and it was believed to be present in the warm ocean off the east coast of China. The Chinese Emperor was seeking the elixir of life (or *"fountain of youth"*) and he commanded his missionaries to bring him back the life-sustaining tonic. To the Emperor's dismay, the mission did not return. Legend states that these Chinese explorers found an island paradise that was too satisfying for them to leave. This island was considered the landmass of *"eternal life."* Legend identifies this place as the prefecture of Okinawa, with its coral base and pristine, clear seas.

Folklore Makes Sense in Science

Many cultures hold similar legends, but the quality and length of life of the inhabitants of Okinawa make this story plausible. Understanding how the habitat of Okinawa promotes health and well-being has been a key focus of anti-aging research for several decades. Whilst one should not believe in *"fairy tales,"* modern researchers have increasingly found that folklore is a great starting point to examine new scientific concepts in natural medicine. In fact, researchers at the National Institutes of Health in the US have used folklore accounts of remedies of natural origin to select botanicals and marine organisms for investigation and research as new treatments. This approach has been found to be especially valuable and productive in the search for new anticancer compounds. Perhaps this is why Okinawan folklore for thousands of years has taught that *"the islands of Okinawa shall cure the world."*

Recorded in the history of Okinawa is the phenomenon of exodus of physicians. Local folklore

45

history holds that physicians and healers left Okinawa when coral was included increasingly in the diet of the local populations. This circumstance was attributed to a precipitous decline in disease, which tended to make the physicians redundant. In addition, popular history refers to enhanced agricultural production when coral was used in agricultural practices as fertilizer and a food supplement (see chapter 4). It should be noted that the Okinawans were a highly educated society and that they meticulously documented their history, and therefore the stories are much more than hearsay.

Precedent, as well as folklore, holds that coral calcium can promote health and well-being in many ways. These claims of benefit range from the prevention of all chronic disease to the successful treatment of cancer, osteoporosis and heart disease. Whilst legend must not be confused with science, the history of the use of coral calcium for health has a long and repeated, successful record. It is logical that things that work sustain themselves over time in human experiences. Whilst the original findings are empiric and considered anecdotal by some scientists, there is an expanding group of modern scholars who swear by the health benefits of coral. Currently, in the United States, there are growing numbers of respected citizens making claims about the medical benefits of coral calcium. (See Chapter 11:Testimonials.)

Makoto Suzuki Speaks

Dr. Makoto Suzuki is the director of the Okinawa Research Center for Longevity Science in Japan. He has repeatedly declared that the most important factor that determines longevity in Okinawa is diet and nutrition. However, many reasons are given for the promotion of health

46

and longevity in Okinawa. At one time the health and longevity of Okinawans were attributed to climatic conditions, and a carefree island mentality. Whilst these and other factors may operate, the special circumstances of health and longevity that are found in the Okinawans are not shared by island dwellers in other locations. The basis of this phenomenon is believed to be the unique role of coral calcium in the food chain (nutrient, life cycle) of the native Okinawans.

Dr. Suzuki has drawn attention to the unique cuisine of the Okinawans which he believes are naturally rich in nutrients. We know that the nutritive value of plant life is a function of the terrain on which it is grown. The infrastructure of the land in Okinawa is based on sea coral and the water supply is mineral-enriched to a major degree as a result of its filtering by coral beds. When water is in contact with coral it takes up a wide range of minerals, marine microbes and other potential nutrients. The beneficial role of the basic coral structure in the nutrition of the Okinawan people seems to be a logical scientific conclusion. After all, we have recognized increasingly the diminished mineral and nutrient depletion of soil as a major factor in reducing the nutritional value of many foods.

Examining Longevity

Longevity is ultimately determined by the time of death. Within this term is the implication of quality of life. This means that longevity is viewed as the length of time that one can live under the most favorable circumstances. The quest for longevity involves the retention of health. In Western society, ill health is often considered to be inevitable with advancing years. Our aim is to move away from this circumstance and toward life expectancy associated with quality of life. In Okinawa health and a long life seem to go together. Why? A question that begs to be answered.

There have been many studies of longevous (long-lived) communities throughout the world. The examination of the social, psychological and physical factors that operate in longevous communities teaches us a great deal. Table 2 highlights several factors that have been proposed as key issues in promoting well-being and a long life.

Table 2
Factors identified in medical research that contribute to longevity. The strength of each factor varies in different populations

FACTOR	COMMENT
Balanced nutrient intake	Foods high in nutrients and essential trace elements.
Trace elements in food	Populations living in areas where minerals are rich in the soil.
Low calorie intake	Relationship in experimental animals. Very strong, evidence in humans.
Dietary restriction	Excessive animal protein is a physiological stress and is associated with excessive saturated fat intake and its sequel – especially cardiovascular disease.

High fiber diets	Variable association with longevity. In non-deprived cultures high fiber diets can be shown to promote health.
Exercise	A common factor for health promotion.
Sociability	Getting along and reducing stress; promotes health and well-being.
Economics	Poor people tend to die young.
Environmental influences	Urban living involves exposure to greater daily stress and pollution.
Education	Intelligence is "environmental" with a genetic component. Intelligence correlates with survival.
Marital status	Being married or in a close supporting relationship promotes health and statistics show a beneficial association between longevity and marriage.
Genetics	Genetic influences on longevity remain unclear but operate to some variable degree.

Of all of the factors listed in Table 2, I believe that the one that stands out in most studies of longevity is the supply of essential trace elements and minerals. The reason for this is not obvious at first sight, but it relates to the fact that basic life processes require essential elements (e.g. calcium, magnesium and zinc etc.) for normal function. I stress the *"essential"* or obligatory nature of minerals for the optimal function of the chemistry of life.

Diet and nutrition figure strongly in anti-aging or longevity theories but food cannot be an efficient source of major nutritive substance, unless it contains the elemental, co-factors for body function. Thus, the supply of abundant elements and minerals underlies the whole concept of the nutritional value of foods. There is strong evidence for my proposals as we examine several communities that live long and healthy lives.

Looking for Longevity Factors

Perhaps the most important clues to understanding the secrets of longevity have come from studies of longevous populations. This observational research was popular forty years ago, but the important findings seem to have been hidden by modern theories involving advanced knowledge of molecular biology. Clearly, contemporary scientists succumb to the perceived necessity to apply modern biotechnology. This circumstance may occur without recognition of the current levels of scientific understanding about life.

There has been a tendency to examine longevity factors by placing them into a perspective that matches the factors with theories of aging. However, the aging process remains incompletely understood and matching anti-aging interventions with hypotheses of aging has been found to be problematic by many scientists. I believe that it is time to stop established precedent by re-examining earlier theories which have been recognized for thousands of years in folklore history and as a consequence of precedent.

One might be impressed by media reports that we are living longer. In actuality, recently human life span has not increased dramatically and in fact lags far behind the experiences of Okinawans and other cultures that exhibit longevity (e.g. Vilacambans, Abkhasians and Hunzukuts). I stress that the *"factor common to all"* of these people seems to be the generous supply of minerals and elements in their environment.

Science Speaks on Minerals and Longevity

Dr. S. Benet published his observation on longevity factors in a book entitled **How to Live to be 100.** (The Dial Press, NY 1976). The book reported by Dr. Benet showed major differences in the dietary patterns of longevous people compared with those with a shorter life span. Similar observations were made by Dr. D. Davis who studied the lifestyle habits and environment of centenarians who live at altitude in the Andes mountains of South America (Davis D, *The Centenarians of the Andes,* Double Day Publishing Co, NY, 1975). Also, Dr. Allen E. Bank, who studied the famous **Hunzas** of Northern Pakistan discovered and reported in his book **Hunza Land**, that their diet was substantially different, and that they ate their food immediately upon harvest or slaughter, and never peeled or skinned their fruits or vegetables. He also noted that they always ate the animal organs, including the delicacy of intestine full of vegetation.

He further noted that they ate several foods that were very high in calcium content, such as soybean flour (330mg/cup), molasses (116mg/tsp), goat's milk (305mg/8oz), kale (450mg/cup), bone meal (610mg/cup), and almonds (572mg/cup). He also quoted Douglas Spies, M.D., a recipient of the **A.M.A. Distinguished Services Award,** who in 1959 in a talk to the members of the American Medical Association said *"All disease is caused by chemicals, and all disease can be cured by chemicals."* (Note: Dr. Hipporates, Father of Medicine declared *"All food is medicine and the best food is the best medicine."*) All the chemicals used by the body are taken in through food. If we only knew enough, all disease could be prevented and could be cured through proper nutrition."

These scientists (Benet and Day) reported independently that people who reached elite, elderly status (greater than 100 years of age) ate a greater amount of vegetables which were particularly high in micronutrients. The same phenomenon has been reported in Okinawans by Dr. Makoto Suzuki during his tenure as a professor at Ryukyu University in Japan. Similar, independent observations have been made in the same population by Yaeko Nishio, a culinary expert from Okinawa.

Hype Transcends Science

The 1970's witnessed great interest in the study of the habitat and lifestyle of populations that exhibited longevity. These studies were aired in the lay press and a fascinating account of this work appeared in the January 1973 edition of *National Geographic* magazine under the title "Search for the Oldest People." Of particular interest were the Hunzas of the mountain regions of Pakistan. So recognized was this phenomenon of longevity that supplement and food manufacturers used the word "Hunza" in the brand name of their products. Products such as the "Hunza colon cleanse" and the "Hunza Health Potion Package" appeared on the nutraceutical market. Even movies loosely based on this culture such as "Shangra La" appeared in theaters. Unfortunately, this circumstance of *"hype"* transcending science served to detract conventional scientists from the important observation of the nutritional factors that were contributory to the longevity of the Hunza population, who are direct descendants of the army of Alexander the great.

The Common Links

Whilst nutrition was identified in 1970's and earlier as a key factor in promoting health and long life, the study of several longevous populations, including the Okinawans, revealed a *"common link"* among these communities. This "common link" was the mineral-enriched habitat in which longevous populations lived. For example, it was recorded that certain water supplies used by these populations contained very high quantities of essential elements of minerals. For example, the Hunza water, known as *"milk of the mountains"* is white and turbid with fine glacial rock. Each quart contains about 20,000 milligrams of calcium, and the Hunzas consume several quarts of this water daily. This means that they are consuming over *100 times the RDA* of calcium, with the only side effects being long life, good health and a dramatic slowing of the aging process. Calcium, magnesium and many vital trace elements are also abundant in the soil and water of several communities of people such as the Abkhasians of Georgia, the Bamas of China and Tibetans. This rich source of essential elements is present in the food chain

53

and these populations tend to eat more vegetables, more fiber and less animal protein than communities with shorter life-spans.

The Okinawan Diet: "Nushi-Gusui"

Okinawan people view food and medicine as synonymous. This was also the view of the Father of Medicine, Dr. Hippocrates, who declared 2,500 years ago that *"all food was medicine and the best food was the best medicine."* The inseparability of food from medicine is reflected in the phrase *"Nuchi-Gusui"* which is used in Okinawa to give thanks for food. In contrast, the term *"Gochi-Soo-Sama"* is a common phrase for giving thanks for meals in mainland Japan. When roughly translated the term *"Nuchi-Gusui"* used by the Okinawans means *"The Life Medicine."* This cultural attitude to food which emphasizes the act of eating to support body structure and function is absent in many Western societies. Certainly, this attitude is inconsistent with the American *"Double Whopper Brain"* and *"Big Gulp Society"* that has created many *"Fast Food Nations."*

Okinawans consume vegetables that are available in other areas of Eastern Asia, but the mineral and micronutrient (element) content of their food is high because it is grown on coral-enriched land fed by water that is filtered and in contact with the rich mineral source of stony corals. A popular local vegetable with special nutrient value is the *"goya."* The goya is an elongated vegetable with a prickly skin. This vegetable is a rich source of antioxidant vitamins B, C and E and it has valuable content of zinc and selenium, which are *"mineral antioxidants."* Antioxidant intake in the diet has been closely linked with anti-aging. Nutritionists have embraced the theories of oxidative damage to tissues, where reactive free radicals contribute to aging.

The most popular staple in the diet of Okinawans is "*firm tofu*" that is precipitate with calcium. The act of "*adding coral calcium*" to tofu has been variably practiced by Okinawans to ensure optimal mineral intake. Tofu is produced from soybeans using special fermentation processes and its universal health benefits have been well recognized (Holt S., *The Soy Revolution*, Dell Publishing, Random House NY, 2000).

The Okinawan tofu is served in generous portions that contain large amounts of vegetable (soy) protein and beneficial quantities of soy Isoflavones (phytoestrogens: genistein, daidzein). In brief, soy consumed as tofu or other fractions can lower blood cholesterol, exert anti-cancer effects (reduction of breast, prostate and colon cancer), reverse osteoporosis, improve renal function and help in preventing obesity. Table 3 traces some of the proposed effects of soy diets on longevity.

Table 3
The potential benefits of soy foods for longevity

CONDITION	EFFECTS OF SOY
Premature death due to:	
Heart disease	Lowers blood cholesterol, antiathero-sclerotic.
Hypertension	Modest lowering of blood pressure.

Cancer	Prevents breast, prostate, colon and other cancers.
Renal failure	Improves renalfunction in comparison to animal protein.
Obesity	Generally low in calories.

Illness in old age due to:

Heart disease	Prevents coronary artery and circulatory disorders.
Skeletal disorders	Soy protein and isoflavones help build bone density and reverse osteoporosis.
Decreased brain function	Phytoestrogens may improve cognitive function, prevent Alzheimer's disease?
Gallstones	Prevents gallstones.
Failing body function in old age	Soy is a good nutritional source with above advantages.

Modified from "The Soy Revolution" Stephen Holt M.D., Dell Publishing, 2000–with permission

Do Not Fear the Healthy Frying Pan

One of the most popular dishes in Okinawa is *"Champuru"* which is made with fried ingredients. This traditional dish has been used since the 14th or 15th Century and it probably originated from the early Chinese settlers on the Okinawan Islands. The term *"Champuru"* means *"to mix"* and this wholesome dish often contains a generous amount of vegetables and tofu. A favored addition to "Champuru" is pork (or "spam" and tuna). The consumption of pork by Okinawans exceeds the rest of Japan but they eat it in specially prepared ways. No part of the pig is spared and it is stated that the Okinawan *"eats very part of the pig except the oink."* (Taiga Uranaka, *Japan Times*, July 17, 2000).

Whilst excessive pork consumption may be linked with high saturated fat intake, the manner in which pork is used in Okinawa is very special. Pigs' blood is used for frying, pigs' feet are consumed with their health given content of collagen and cartilage and much of the pork is boiled to remove excess fat. In contrast, pork consumption in Western society is often in the form of salted bacon, sausages and ham. This Western way of eating pork is associated with cardiovascular disease and stroke.

High salt intake in Japan, as in America, has been associated by medical officials with a high incidence of hypertension, stroke and gastric cancer among certain populations. However in Japan the salt consumption is higher than in America which also has a much higher incidence of heart disease. This is consistent with other long living cultures, the Hunzas, for example, who put *"handfuls"* of salt into their food and drinks, and rarely have heart disease. This indicates that medical officials are wrong about harm done by salt consumption. A recent study by Dr. Michael Alderman, chairman of epidemiology at the Albert Einstein School of medicine in New York and president of the American Society of Hypertension states *"The lower the sodium the worse off you are."* He found that, overall, a 1,000 milligram increase in dietary salt was associated with a 10% reduction in mortality, and a 10,000 mg daily (one teaspoon) increase provides a 400% reduction in heart attacks. He states that salt restriction triggers heart attacks by elevating blood levels of *renin*, a kidney hormone that helps regulate blood pressure and the excretion of sodium. Too much renin leads to too much *angiotensin II*, a related compound that causes constriction of the coronary arteries. Thus, the concept that "too much salt is bad for you" is another *medical myth* in America.

Coral Calcium Meets Soy

It is apparent that coral calcium contains general amounts of calcium and magnesium which forms *"salts."* However, other essential trace elements such as zinc and copper form salts and these are found in sea water and coral. Sea water contains concentrations of elements that are often higher than levels found in the tissues of humans. Although the elements of the ocean are more concentrated, the proportions of the various salts are similar to those found in animal tissues. When seawater is evaporated completely a residue remains that is about three quarters sodium chloride by weight. The remainder is composed of minerals of many types (more than seventy different elements). Traditional Japanese cuisine has used this kind of *"ash residue"* of marine origin to make tofu. The residue is prepared from sea water in a way that removes much of the sodium chloride (equivalent to table salt). This kind of preparation is called *"nigari"* which is used to solidify soy bean curd or tofu by traditional methods. The nutritional benefits of soy are combined with a rich depot of minerals in this special way of preparing tofu. Coral calcium can be used in a similar way to add to tofu with a resulting nutritional mixture of soy protein, antioxidant phyto-chemicals and essential minerals. This traditional culinary approach achieves many of the factors that we know are associated with health and longevity. These factors include vegetable sources of protein, relatively low calorie intake and abundant mineral supplies.

The Okinawan Secret?

For many years Okinawans have used coral in inventive ways and even when not added to cuisine, its habitual presence enriches the environment largely through its presence in water. For many years, scientists and researchers attributed longevity in Okinawa Prefecture to the climate and diet of the people, but in the 1950's Professor Jun Kobayashi revealed his "groundbreaking" work that showed *"a direct relationship between the 'hard water' that is consumed by Okinawans and their long and healthy life span."* The work of Professor Kobyashi was published in *The Sokai Journal of Okinawa* under the loosely translated title, *"The Secret of Health and Longevity in Okinawa, Where Many People Live to an Advanced Age and Where the Incidence of All Diseases is Low."*

Soft and Hard Water

So vital is water that humans can survive only a few days without it. We have learned that water has a unique chemistry which makes it the ideal basis to support life forms, including the biological mass of the human body. The best selling author John Langone draws attention to the phenomenon of *"dying water"* in his book *Our Endangered Earth* (Little, Brown and Co., 1992). Without fresh water there is no life and despite the absolute requirement of water for health, society does relatively little to protect itself from "dying water" that is changed to an unhealthy composition or polluted by humankinds' interventions. Society has focused much attention on making water potable but we may have been using false logic in some of our approaches to create an optimal domestic water supply.

The importance of Professor Kobayashi's work on *"Hard Water in Okinawa and Longevity"* has been underestimated in Western medicine and nutrition. The natural fresh water of Okinawa has been identified as containing a high mineral content because it is filtered through coral remains where it picks up vital minerals and elements in a form that is readily utilized in biochemical mechanisms of life. Few scientists would doubt the potential benefits of water with high mineral content but this quality of water has been underutilized as a medical treatment or disease preventive. Examination of disease and survival statistics in Japan shows clearly that the mineral content of water in Okinawa has material health advantages over the *"soft water"* (mineral deficient) that is consumed on mainland Japan, and in many Western communities.

Volcanic Soil Meets Coral

It is clear that the geological evolution of Okinawa and its adjacent islands affects the environmental availability of minerals. These Ryukyu islands are composed of about 60 land masses of variable size that form an arc in the ocean, spanning several hundred miles. The largest land masses are volcanic in origin with raised profiles, but the coral islands tend to be flat. A unique feature of this geography, that may account for even more abundance of various minerals, is the *"proximity of coral reefs to volcanic material."* Volcanic material forms soils that are exceedingly rich in trace elements, resulting in an even greater source of minerals that are incorporated into Okinawan coral. Thus the coral from Okinawa is dramatically chemically different from all other corals. In addition, its marine microbes are specific to the islands of Okinawa, and are not found in other corals. Thus Okinawan coral is uniquely different from all other corals.

"Inconvenience" of Hard Water: Key Health Hazards

Many communities have tried to soften water. I believe that the modern tendency of water softening is a great threat to health. *"Hard water"* is naturally high in calcium and magnesium, which are the two most abundant elements in marine coral calcium! When domestic water is hard it tends to reduce detergent and soap actions and it can clog pipes and parts of domestic appliances. In addition, washing clothes in hard water can cause salt deposition with gray spots and it leaves a film on dishes and pots. These minor inconveniences have led to the *"folly"* of softening domestic water supplies.

Soft water has a higher content of sodium, which is very unhealthy when consumed, and it is produced in many areas of the world by removing calcium and magnesium from water. I believe that the evidence for the health benefits of minerals or elements, such as calcium and magnesium, is so strong that *"water softening"* must be regarded as a *"major public health concern."* All of the long living and relatively disease-free cultures of the world have hard water. Softening involves robbing health-enhancing calcium and magnesium whilst adding unhealthy sodium! Using soft water for drinking or cooking results in an unwanted extra source of sodium in the diet.

The negative health implications of soft water have been *"played down"* in western society for reasons that are not clear. Not only does soft water supply excess, unwanted sodium that is harmful to our diet, it is much more effective at dissolving heavy metals which have significant toxicities. Although lead pipes have been replaced in modern construction by copper pipes, soft water tends to be efficient at dissolving toxic heavy metals. Soft water dissolves more lead, mercury and cadmium than hard water, which also tends to precipitate out toxic elements. These elements in small quantities are toxic to many cellular functions, affect brain function and impair immunity. Well-controlled scientific studies have shown that deaths from heart disease are lower in areas where the drinking water is hard. The presence of calcium and magnesium in hard water are believed to play a protective role against heart disease (see *The Natural Way to a Healthy Heart* by S. Holt M.D., M. Evans Publishers Inc., NY, NY, 1999). The domestic *"inconvenience of hard water"* is a small price to pay for health benefits of mineral-enriched hard water.

Okinawan Coral Changes the Environment

Calcium is available in many different forms or foods in our diet but we know that calcium is most active in body chemistry in its ionized form. Coral calcium contains ionized calcium, which carries a positive electrical charge (see Chapter 4). When coral calcium is added to average *"softened water"* it transforms water into a slightly alkaline drink and it buffers and *removes chlorine and fluorine* (which is often added to tap water with dubious evidence of benefit). Some nutritionists have likened the mineral content of coral-enriched water to certain nurturing body fluids such as amniotic fluid and they have stressed its potential antioxidant qualities.

Coral calcium in Okinawa and some adjacent islands assists in the purification and detoxification of the domestic water supply. The coral enriches the potable water with calcium, magnesium, trace elements and a variety of less well characterized elements from the oceans. Coral calcium has been used to raise the pH (alter the acidity or alkalinity of water) and it produces an alkalinizing effect. Some practitioners of alternative medicine believe that alkalinity induced in this way has powers to restore health, treat infection, suppress cancer and promote immunity.

Popular Misunderstandings of Coral in Water

Coral calcium was first introduced to Western culture when it was brought to Europe by the Spanish explorers about 500 years ago. The world's oldest drugstores in Spain, which today are historic monuments, have clay pots on their shelves labeled *"Coral Calcium, Okinawa Japan."* Literature written by doctors of the day told of miraculous cures. By the turn of the 20th Century, the consumption of coral had spread to mainland Japan, where currently there are about 17 million users. Today there are millions of consumers in China, Russia, Britain, France and Sweden. When coral calcium was brought to the Western communities as a *"modern"* dietary supplement in the 1970's, much misunderstanding was propagated by marketing companies. There is a *naïve notion* that when coral calcium is added to water it should dissolve completely. I am often asked about this circumstance, but the answer is obvious. If coral were soluble in water completely there would be no coral reefs in the oceans!

The reason why this question is asked often relates to the popular use of coral sand in tea bags, which are merely added to water and the water is then consumed. Whilst coral calcium tea bags can import desirable properties to water, such as the transfer of important marine microbes, taking coral calcium in this manner is far less desirable then consuming the whole coral in powder or capsule form. Tea bag coral is more of a gimmick, as the user is only benefiting from about 2% of the marine nutrients that dissolve and the consumer, unless told, is almost unaware that he is consuming coral water, than a valuable way of obtaining the full benefits of coral calcium when it is consumed in its whole format, resulting in the consumption of over 50 times as much mineral nutrients. Also, the marine coral that is totally consumed is rich in the required nutrient, magnesium, as well as richer in all other nutrients.

Part of the sales gimmick of some forms of coral calcium is to add substances that rapidly change the pH (alkalinity or acidity) of water. Emptying capsules of coral calcium and testing water immediately is neither scientific nor a reliable measure of the benefits of marine coral.

Fossilized coral that has been washed up on to beaches has lost some of its mineral content by weathering and it may be dried and finely powdered to make a quick change of water pH. In addition, some commercially available coral calcium products have calcium added in hydroxide forms to increase alkalinity. Also, fossilized coral contains less than 1% magnesium, whereas marine coral has about 12% magnesium, which balances the 24% calcium for a perfect biological 2:1 calcium/magnesium ratio. Because of this lack of magnesium in fossilized coral, magnesium compounds are often added, resulting in a substantial dilution of the coral. After studying many types of coral supplements, I have concluded that marine coral, not fossilized coral, taken in whole format is obviously the most ideal way to consume coral calcium for health.

As a result of competition, those selling fossilized coral mislead the public into thinking that because they remove their coral from the beaches they are not harming the coral reefs, implying that those *"mining"* the marine coral must be harming the reefs. The truth is that the *"harvesting"* of the marine coral is done under the strict supervision off the Japanese Government who enforce, by jail incarceration, if the slightest damage occurs. In reality, the deposition of the coral sands (coral calcium) at the base of the reef actually inhibits the growth of the coral reefs. Once this sand is removed by harvesting, the reefs flourish. Thus, harvesting marine coral calcium is not only beneficial to man but to the coral reefs as well.

Despite the deficiencies, both tea bag coral and fossilized coral consumption has led to remarkable health testimonials, although not as many as the consumption of marine coral. This is due to the *"microbe factor"* (explained in detail in the next paragraph). In addition there are many other factors that make coral calcium of marine origin more ideal for health. I prefer coral that is used in vegetable capsules or at least capsules that are made to dissolve at the right time to provide the best circumstances for mineral absorption. The practice of breaking capsules and adding the contents to water is unnecessary, except in circumstances where some people cannot readily swallow capsules.

Microbes or bacillus are defined as any genus of rod-shaped bacteria that occur in chains, produce spores and are active only in the presence of oxygen and water. Although some microorganisms are destroyed in the process of drying, this process is not per se lethal to microorganisms. The addition of water can spring them back to life. Microbes can be found living in all living animals and plants. Of course most microbes can live off of plants and food, and are best known for their ability to *"spoil"* the food. Actually *spoiling food is a form of digestion*. Thus, spoiled food is pre-digested by the microbes. This is probably the reason that most of the animal kingdom, including humans, have substantial numbers of microbes in their intestines. The strong acid in the stomach can not break down all food, especially complex carbohydrates. However, the microbes in the intestine living off of these foods, do indeed break them down and make them available for absorption by the small intestine. Also, the rod-like shape, allows the microbes to penetrate deep into the *"finger-like villi,"* 5 million lining the intestine, where they can easily be absorbed by 1) *facilitated diffusion* (glucose combines with a carrier substance which is soluble in the lipid layer of the cell membrane), 2) *osmosis* (the movement of water molecules and dissolved solids through semi-permeable cell membranes from an area of high concentration to an area of low concentration), 3) *filtration* (movement of solvents and dissolved substances across semipermeable cell membranes by mechanical pressure, usually high pressure to low pressure), 4) *dialysis* (separation of small molecules from large molecules by semi-permeable membrane) and 5) *pinocytosis* (or "cell drinking" where the liquid nutrient attracted to the surface of the cell membrane is engulfed). As a result, the *"microbes are crucial to life."* Fortunately, most of the hundreds of non- marine microbes found in the human intestine were transferred by the mother. Some animals, like the baby elephant, have to eat their mother's excrement just to get the needed microbes.

The genera of bacteria that are found in the intestinal tract are: Bacteroides (22 species, non-sporing rods), Clostridium (61 species, heat-resistant spore-forming rods),

Citrobacter (2 species, lactose-fermenting rods), Enterobacter (2 rods, ferment glucose and lactose), Escherichia (one specie, rods), Lactobacillus (27 species, non-sporing rods employed in the production of fermented milks), Proteus (5 species, aerobic rods that hydrolyze urea), Pseudomonas, 29 species, most important bacteria in spoilage of meats, poultry, eggs and seafoods), Salmonella (1800 species that ferment sugars and glucose), Shigella (4 species, aerobic, like pollutuon), Staphylococcus (3 species, coagulate blood, also common in nasal cavities) and Streptococcus (21 species).

Salt greater than 1% can cross the cell membranes of most bacterium by osmosis, which results in growth inhibition and possibly death of the microbes. Everyone is also familiar with the preservation of meat by *"salting,"* which kills or inhibits the bacteria. Thus large quantities of salt in the intestinal tract, which occur when large quantities of nutrients have been digested (hydrochloric acid from the stomach reacting with the sodium bicarbonate from the pancreas produces salt in the duodenum), can kill the microbes, thereby inhibiting nutrient absorption by the body, especially when large amounts of nutrients have been injested.

On the contrary, *"marine microbes,"* such as those found in coral calcium, thrive in high salt environments. Also because of their original salty marine environment, as well as their calcium magnesium and mineral environment, the marine microbes have no difficulty assisting the body to absorb high quantities of these minerals, especially when the intestine is saline, resulting from the consumption of large amounts of mineral nutrients. These same salts, however, incapacitate the natural microbes in the intestinal tract, thereby inhibiting nutrient absorption. Thus, the coral marine microbes resolve this problem, dramatically increasing the absorption of the nutrients by the body.

Those people using a small sachet teabag that allows only a tiny amount of coral to dissolve in the liquid in which they are placed, and those using fossilized coral, still get some benefits from the marine microbes, hence the testimonials. Also, these testimonies emanating from the small intake of nutrients are nothing short of astounding. The reason for this success is that when the teabag or the fossilized coral is placed in a liquid the microbes come to life and are consumed when the liquid is drank. These microbes can then latch on to nutrients already in the duodenum and pull them into the body resulting in health benefits. Consumption of marine coral, on the other hand, allows the *"total nutrient content of the coral"* to be consumed as well, and therefore provides far greater health benefits, leading to more testimonials. The bottom line is that all coral from Okinawa has fantastic health benefits, but the *marine coral is far superior*.

I believe that there are certain elements that serve a health purpose when added to coral (e.g. Rubidium, Vanadium, Boron, Silver and Nickel). I have summarized examples of what I believe to be crucial trace metals in Table 4. My recommendations on the health benefit of certain elements may tend to differ somewhat from classic teaching and I am not recommending anything more than very small trace amounts of metals that have underexplored health benefits. My belief in the benefit of certain trace metals that are not popular as supplements comes from my research on populations where longevity is the norm. For example, the native Hunzas drink up to 30 cups of tea on a daily basis (the tea is made from the milk of the mountains glacial water that is loaded with minerals, including about 20,000 milligrams of calcium per quart) which they flavor with handfuls of rock salt that contain ever more abundant minerals and trace elements, many of which are listed in Table 4. They also like to add a paddy of butter to each cup of tea. It should be noted that this salt consumption, along with the calcium consumption, vastly exceeds the RDA allowables.

The Hunzas form a very interesting precedent for the safety of abundant mineral intake. It is also interesting to note that most Hunza men prefer to have children when they are more mature, in their 70s when they are capable of carrying heavy loads many miles over mountain passes. Hunzas with their mineral-rich rock salt, aggregate and Okinawans with their mineral-rich coral calcium, form youthful, energetic, disease-free people who live to a ripe old age. Whilst, Western physicians who treat human patients have not often recognized the importance of mineral and metal supplements, veterinarians have taken a lead with our pets and other domestic animals. Whilst horse and dog food contains tens of nutrient supplements, much human food is quite depleted in these same life-sustaining nutrients. If anyone questions this logic, then I invite him to analyze the contents of popular junk food that accounts for the highest amount of calorie intake in many Western diets. Even baby food is lucky to have up to only 10 nutrients added, while most dog food has over 50.

Furthermore, we shall learn that coral calcium taken in capsules is not "*designed*" to provide all the necessary dietary intake of calcium and a calcium-rich diet is advised along with coral supplements (hence the term "supplement"). This is the way the environment works in Okinawa!

In summary, *marine coral* harvested from the sea bed is the most ideal type of coral for use in dietary supplements. It has a composition that is closest in its organic, mineral and element content to that of the exoskeleton of the living reef coral. It is best taken in a particulate preparation, which is placed in vegetable capsules with ideal dissolution (dissolving) characteristics.

Table 4
Some Crucial Trace Metals

Metal	Biochemical Purpose
Boron	Needed in trace amounts for calcium uptake and healthy bones, and for the maintenance of normal levels of estrogen and testosterone in the blood.
Bismuth	Kills the bacterium helicobacter pylori, which is proven to be the *"cause of peptic ulcers."*
Chromium	Essential in the manufacture of cholesterol, fats and protein and maintains proper blood sugar levels and is therefore crucial in deterring diabetes.
Cesium	The largest and *most alkaline metal*, which, once inside the human cell, cannot leave, thereby neutralizing the acids which "cause" the degenerative diseases, such as cancer, heart disease, arthritis, etc.

Cobalt	Necessary for *the production of the thyroid hormone*, and is a crucial component of vitamin-B-12 whichhelps prevent anemia.
Copper	An important component of hundreds of human enzymes which help maintain the body's elasticity (youth), especially in the skin (*preventing wrinkles*) and in the cartilage and muscles and thus, helps to prevent aneurysms, arthritis, Cerebral Palsy, hernias, etc.. Also restores color to greying hair and is crucial for iodine utilization.
Germanium	Acts as a carrier for oxygen, similar to hemoglobin, and is therefore excellent at *tissue oxygenation* to help preventviral infections.
Iodine	Crucial component of the thyroid hormone thyroxin, which regulates heart rate, body temperature, digestion, general metabolism, body weight, the nervous system and reproductive system.
Lithium	Helps to *dissolve kidney stones*. Helps to control criminal behavior and depression. Lithium deficiency can leadto manic depression, reproductive failure, and reduced growth rate.

Manganese	Crucial component of many hormones, enzymes and proteins and is an *activator for cartilage* and bone development. Manganese deficiency can lead to deafness, asthma, carpal tunnel syndrome and birth defects.
Molybdenum	Constituent of many crucial enzymes including Aldehyde oxidase, sulfite oxidase, and xanthine oxidase.
Praseodymium	Enhances the proliferation of normal cell growth, and in laboratory tests has doubled the life of some species of animals.
Rubidium	The second largest and second most alkaline metal, which, once inside the human cell, cannot leave, thereby *neutralizing the acids* which cause the degenerative diseases such as cancer, heart disease, arthritis, etc.
Selenium	Selenium is the strongest metal antioxidant: it prevents cellular fats and lipids from going rancid and producing age spots and liver spots. It also helps *to prevent heart palpitations*, liver cirrhosis, sclerosis, cystic fibrosis, muscular dystrophy, multiple sclerosis, Alzheimer's, cancer, etc.
Silicon	Silicon helps keep fingernails and hair

	from becoming brittle while more than doubling the collagen in bone growth.
Tin	Helps prevent both *hearing and hair loss* while also helping to prevent cancer.
Vanadium	*Enhances DNA synthesis* and stimulates blood sugar oxidation helping to prevent diabetes.
Yttrium	Enhances the proliferation of *normal cell growth*, and in laboratory tests has doubled the life of some species of animals.
Zinc	Required for protein synthesis and collagen formation necessary for a healthy heart and healthy lungs, and also *promotes a healthy immune system* and the healing of wounds.

Reported Benefits of Coral Calcium from Okinawa

I have stressed that our *scientific knowledge* about the health benefits of coral calcium *remains incomplete*, and new information is constantly being added. For example, Swedish researchers recently discovered that coral calcium contains microbes, as previously discussed in this chapter, specific to Okinawa. They claim that these microbes are responsible for the rapid and complete absorption of the mineral nutrients, as thousands of microbes in the human intestine are credited with assisting absorption of nutrients in the human body. They point to the fact that *unhealthy blood* with the oxygen depleted red cells stacked (rouleau) and the whiter cells overactive in the presence of large quantities of uric acid crystals, immediately (within minutes) upon the consumption of coral calcium, becomes *healthy blood* with the red cells spherical and full of oxygen, the white cells spherical and at rest and most of the uric acid dissolved and missing. Medical researchers have also discovered that the Okinawan centenarian has the arteries of a child. Also, users of coral calcium have reported many health benefits including relief from arthritis, osteoporosis, inflammatory diseases, cardiovascular disorders and anti-cancer benefits. Contemporary authors on the subject of the health benefits of coral calcium have reported relief from arthritic pain, allergies, reflux symptoms from hiatal hernia, gout, colitis and, other digestive problems. In addition, beneficial reducts in blood sugar and blood pressure have been proposed with reports of weight loss, relief from fibromyalgia and chronic fatigue (Owen BL, *Why Calcium?* Health Digest Books, Cannon Beach, OR). In his book *Fossil Stony Coral Minerals and Their Nutritional Application,* Dr. Bruce Halstead M.D. stresses the benefits of mineralized water for cardiovascular health and highlights the power and versatility of coral calcium (stony corals) for disease treatment and prevention.

Using Coral in Surgery

Coral is also very much like human bone and the body does not reject it, and it is conducive to allowing new bone growth. In Germany, surgeons will pack the cracks and holes in the broken bones of the elderly with a coral paste made from coral calcium and water. Within three weeks the coral is displaced with new bone growth. James Tobin in the Detroit News writes that "*because of a gift from the sea, coral calcium,*

Christian Groth is swimming again." The coral rests snuggly inside the femur (thigh bone) of his right leg, just above the knee. It fills a hole the size of a large marble, replacing a benign tumor that was making it harder and harder for Chris, 14, to play the sports he loves. If you use a powerful microscope to compare the coral to Chris' bone, you could not tell the difference. "Chris is one of the first people in Metro Detroit to have a bone repaired with sea coral and *is doing everything,*" said his doctor, Ronald Irwin, an orthopedic oncologist affliliated with the Beaumint Hospital, Royal Oak. *"It looks good,"* Irwin said, *"he'll ski this year!"*

The May issue of the New England Journal of Medicine, 2001, wrote about the *"bionic thumb."* Doctor Charles Vacanti at the University of Massachusetts re-created a thumb for Paul Murcia who had lost his thumb in a machine accident. First a small sample on bone from the patient's arm bone was cultured to multiply. Then a sea coral scaffold was sculpted into the shape of the missing thumb bone, and then implanted into Murcia's thumb. The patient's own bone cells, grown in the lab, were then injected onto the scaffold. The bone cells grew a blood supply and the coral scaffold slowly melted away leaving a new living thumb bone. The doctors predict that eventually all that will be left will be a thumb bone with healthy bone cells and no coral. Twenty-eight months after the surgery the patient is able to use his thumb relatively normally and the doctors say that the experiment in tissue engineering using the coral is working.

CHAPTER 4

Coral Calcium Contents

Different Forms of Coral

The widespread confidence in the health benefits of coral calcium from Okinawa has led to an emerging coral mining industry involving more than a dozen companies supplying thousands of distributors on a worldwide basis. In my writings and media appearances, I have stated that *"all Okinawan coral is good coral, with some coral being better than others,"* as a consequence of my research on the link between minerals and health. However, certain forms of coral from Okinawa and adjacent islands differ in their mineral content and residual organic contents from the ocean. The Okinawans grade the coral based on "magnesium content," the higher the magnesium content, the better the grade. It will become apparent that marine coral collected from the ocean bed is the most desirable form when used as a dietary supplement for health.

Coral can be mined on the seashores, an underwater vacuuming operation overseen by the Japanese government. It is interesting to note that damaging the coral in any way leads to incarceration, and that after the coral sands are removed from the base of the coral, the coral flourishes. This coral contains about 12% magnesium with 24% calcium, the perfect biological ratio, and is considered to be the highest grade. Coral can also be collected on beaches in a fossilized form. In fact, much use of coral calcium has involved this type of fossilized material. This weathered coral usually contains less than 1% magnesium and is considered to be the lowest grade. Crude fossilized coral is ground and heated with variable applications of disinfectants. Bleach is sometimes used in an inappropriate manner to *"purify"* fossilized coral. I believe that *"bleached coral"* may not contain a number of organic or bio-organic remnants, such as the nutrient absorbing microbes, that may enhance the bioactive role of coral and it can also alter the natural ionization of coral minerals.

Whilst the term "coral calcium" stresses the presence of calcium within this remedy of natural origin, it must be emphasized that stony corals contain more than seventy different, valuable minerals or elements that have been proven to promote health. Coral collected from the seabed, *"marine coral"* that has been shed from the coral reef in a natural manner, has a greater bioactive composition than fossilized coral; and as previously stated, it is naturally rich in magnesium.

The ratio of calcium to magnesium in *"marine coral"* approaches 2 to 1, which is the ideal ratio of administration of these minerals for nutritional support of body structure and function. In contrast, *"fossilized coral"* collected on the beaches is somewhat deficient in magnesium and other trace nutrients. Some nutrient companies add magnesium to achieve the desired 2 to 1 balance of calcium to magnesium. In simple terms the coral that contains the most nutrients, the least damaged in processing, and that most resembles the coral of the living reef, is *"marine coral,"* and this form of coral is to be preferred with the caveat that *"all coral is good, but some is much superior to others,"* at least in vital micronutrient components.

Mineral Analysis of Coral Calcium

Dr. Bruce Halstead has reported several analyses of fossil stony coral samples in his book entitled *Fossil Stony Coral Minerals and Their Nutritional Application* (Health Digest Publishing Co, Cannon Beach, OR). In his reports on fossilized coral the most common components of coral calcium are calcium and magnesium that occur as salts with carbonic acid (carbonates). In fossilized coral, as has been discussed, these carbonates of calcium and magnesium occur in about a 12 to 1 ratio (86% calcium carbonate versus 7.5 % magnesium carbonate). The Japanese believe that this is because the less stable magnesium carbonate disintegrates over time due to weathering. In contrast, the recently harvested marine coral has a higher magnesium content with some samples approaching the biologically perfect 2 to 1 calcium to magnesium ratio (implying that Mother Nature knew what it was doing when it made coral calcium). This is a fundamental advantage for the use of marine coral as a nutraceutical.

Table 5 lists the parts per million of the main elements found in fossilized corals. A detailed breakdown of the mineral profile of coral is shown in Table 5. It is apparent that almost every natural element known to man finds its way into stony coral over the many years of growth of the reefs. The chemical analysis is always expressed as whole rock analyses which, if accurate, should add up to about 99% with the 1% balance being composed of trace elements (see Table 6b). The elements are expressed as oxides with the loss on ignition (the weight loss when heated to 1,000 degrees Centigrade) representing the gasses lost upon heating; water, carbon, nitrogen and sulfur.

Table 5: Major Elements Found in Marine Coral Calcium
– certified "whole rock" analyses, R. Barefoot.

Assay	Percent	PPM Metal
Silicon Dioxide	3.92	18,318
Aluminum Oxide	0.32	1,693
Calcium Oxide	33.60	240,000
Magnesium Oxide	18.90	114,000
Sodium Oxide	0.42	3,360
Strontium Oxide	0.33	2,770
Iron Oxide	0.14	979
Loss on Ignition	41.3	
Total Majors	**98.93%**	

NB: Loss on ignition is the total of water, carbon, nitrogen, sulfur

Table 6: Trace Elements Found in Coral Calcium
-certified "trace" analyses by R. Barefoot
*-adapted from Bhalstead, M.D. 1999

Elements	Result (ppm)	Elements	Result (ppm)
Aluminum	1693	Manganese	20
Silver	7	Molybdenum	<1
Arsenic	trace	Niobium	<1
Barium	10	Nickel	7
Boron	1	Phosphorus	280
Bismuth	4	Potassium	830
Cadmium	trace	Lead	trace
Cobalt	11	Rubidium	20
Chromium	80	Antimony	<2
Cesium	20	Selenium	14
Copper	23	Strontium	2770
Iron	979	Yttrium	3

79

Iodine	9	Vanadium	20
Hafnium	<1	Tungsten	0.1
Mercury	0.01	Zinc	16
Lanthanum	2	Zirconium	<1
*Bromine	0.14	*Osmium	<0.2
*Deuterium	150	*Palladium	0.025
*Dysprosium	0.18	*Platinum	<0.03
*Erbium	5.19	*Praseodymium	2.73
*Europium	<0.1	*Rhenium	<0.2
*Gadolinium	0.094	*Rhodium	<0.02
*Gallium	0.692	*Ruthenium	0.081
*Germanium	0.191	*Samarium	<0.05
*Gold	<0.05	*Scandium	0.049
*Holmium	0.091	*Sulfur	1780
*Indium	<0.06	*Tantalum	<0.01
*Iridium	<0.04	*Tellurium	<0.02
*Lithium	0.66	*Tin	0.198
*Lutetium	0.78		

Elemental Forms Within Coral

Whilst the comprehensive mineral content of coral calcium is impressive, the importance of the chemical form of these elements with coral must be appreciated. Many of the elements are present in a form that is well absorbed by the body. In this form these elements can be made readily available for their vital role in body chemistry. The role of minerals in body functions is summarized in a simplified manner in Table 7.

Minerals act on body functions by tending to oppose one another in a harmonious form of chemical balance. Thus, there is a situation of chemical antagonism among minerals which is part of the body's reciprocal and harmonious function. This is what the 19th century scientist Claude Bernard referred to as part of "the harmony of life."

Table 7
A Simple Overview of the Importance of
Minerals in Body Structures and Functions.

Essential <u>major</u> minerals include calcium, magnesium, potassium, sodium and chloride. There are many other essential trace minerals. Although trace minerals are essential they are required in small quantities in the diet.

- Specific role in energy production and cellular structure and function
- Absolute requirement for bone and tooth development and maintenance
- Major components of enzyme systems that drive chemical reactions in the body
- Important function in nerve transmission and muscle function, especially cardiac muscle
- Central role in protein synthesis, hemoglobin synthesis and function and hormone production

The absorption and utilization of minerals by the human body is dependent on a number of biological and chemical factors. The most important issue is to achieve a regular and optimal intake of major and minor essential minerals that support the chemistry of life. The chemical form in which minerals are presented to the body is a key factor in their efficient utilization in the chemistry of life. If minerals are presented in a solution in water (in their ionic form), they are used more efficiently in body processes. If coral calcium is added to pure water a substantial proportion of its valuable content of minerals becomes ionic. This situation contrasts with minerals taken in dry powder or other supplement forms (e.g. tablets) where less of the minerals may be available for use by the body (bio-available). It should be noted that within seconds of entering the stomach, over 99% of the coral becomes ionized (test run by Barefoot using stomach acid on coral calcium) and ready for absorption by the body.

The Importance of Chelated Minerals

Dr. Bruce Halstead MD has drawn attention to the importance of minerals in a *"chelated"* form for efficient use by the body. The process of chelation of minerals occurs in nature where <u>organic</u> substances are bound to metal ions (metallic minerals). The term *"chelation"* is derived from the Greek word *"chele"* which refers to the claw of a crab. The chemical circumstance of chelation is like a tight, pincer binding of metals (held in "crab's claws"). This process of chelation is sometimes known as *"bio-inorganic binding."* The chelation process tends to form a stable complex with the metal ion, by blocking reactive sites on the metal itself.

This chelation process occurs to a major degree in coral calcium, according to the chelation therapy expert Bruce Halstead M.D. The act of chelation ("crab claw" binding of metals) is a very important process in nature for the incorporation of vital metals (calcium, magnesium etc.) in body chemistry. Studies have shown that chelated metals are absorbed and used by the body in a more efficient manner than *"plain"* minerals or elements. This is because the chelated mineral has a rod-like form, the perfect shape to penetrate the fingerlike villi which line the small intestine. In fact, the process of chelation therapy in humans has become a highly valued technique in alternative medicine for removing unwanted metals and treating a variety of diseases. The process of producing enhanced chelation of minerals are used in some manufacturing processes of coral calcium and these stony coral minerals have been reported by Dr. Halstead to be more effective in clinical terms. Marine coral has a greater percentage composition of chelated minerals than fossilized coral, which is another reason to prefer the freshly harvested coral from the ocean.

Antagonism Among Minerals

There is a well-known circumstance of *"interference"* or *"antagonism"* between different minerals that determines the use of minerals by the body. Each element or mineral belongs on an *"electrochemical"* gradient, which accounts for their reactivities in nature. Some elements are highly reactive with their surroundings because of their *"charges"* (electrochemical properties) and this means that excesses of one mineral can put the balance of minerals in nature into a state of *"imbalance."*

It is well known that excesses of one mineral can inhibit the important actions of another mineral. Whilst some scientists question the importance of this balance, it is clear that coral calcium of natural origin is derived from *"life forms"* (the coral polyps) that secrete and elaborate the stony coral in a completely natural manner, using the balance of nature. I believe that this natural origin of balanced mineral content of coral makes it advantageous as a valuable, micronutrient support system for the human body.

Understanding the Production of Coral Calcium
As a Nutraceutical

I have mentioned repeatedly that I believe that marine-based coral is more desirable as a health giving dietary supplement than fossilized stony coral. Some individuals who are very concerned about the environment should understand that coral calcium can be harvested from the land (fossilized coral) or from the ocean bed at the base of the coral reef. Clearly, mining fossilized coral has little effect on the environment. However, land based coral contains a relatively large amount of plain sand (silica) which serves little nutritional benefit. In contrast, marine-based coral from the ocean floor can be collected not only with ecological safety, but its collection can actually help the environment.

Marine coral sand is the *"droppings"* that normally occur from the edges of the coral reefs, over a period of decades. These droppings are the result of normal wave action, which can fracture small terminal elements of the coral reef. In addition, the coral-munching fish deposits some of the marine coral sand. Removing the particulate coral from the seabed around the reef is like *"pruning roses,"* in a simple sense. We have learned that the coral reefs associated with underwater volcanic structures, such as found off the shores of Okinawa, grow sideways to cover pits produced by volcanoes on the seabed. Therefore, removing the marine coral calcium droppings around the reef provide a clear, uninterrupted pathway for expansion and new growth of the reef, as well as making them extremely mineral-rich.

Many commercial companies have promoted coral

calcium from Okinawa as though it is all the same material. However, the harvesting of marine bed coral calcium is much more difficult and costly than merely collecting fossilized coral from beach mines. This fossilized coral has undergone thousands, if not millions, of years of erosion, losing most of its magnesium content and much of its trace metal nutrient content. Also, because of the hype generated by coral calcium testimonials, numerous, unscrupulous entrepreneurs are harvesting coral from other locations around the world (this coral does not have the desired marine microbes), but telling their customers that it comes from Okinawa. Some even go so far as to blend their coral with Okinawan coral so that they can make the claim that it comes from Okinawa. Therefore, interested consumers of food grade coral must be aware of *"cheap"* coral products sold as food supplements. Some of these cheaper products are not only fossilized coral, but they are coral that is *"cut"* with chalk or other inexpensive forms of inorganic minerals. Thus, the consumer must be aware of the raw material harvesting of coral in the product that they use. Whilst I support the use of Okinawan coral for health, it is a fact that marine-based coral has far greater health-giving potential than fossilized coral.

My Studies of Marketed Coral Calcium

In my studies of the selection of different types of coral, I have learned that careful selection of a suitable grade material is necessary. Therefore, I was horrified to find some commercial types of coral calcium that were less than 10% coral calcium. This practice has emerged in the manufacture of some types of coral calcium capsules. The addition of inert magnesium or calcium should be disclosed by manufacturers on their labels. The public should look for a label that declares a minimum of *"1,000 milligrams of coral calcium"* content (from Okinawa) in a daily dose, preferably "marine coral." Many of the diluted versions have less than 500 milligrams of coral calcium per daily dose.

As mentioned earlier, marine-based or fossilized coral calcium does not alone provide enough magnesium to meet recommended magnesium levels for health. This is why, I have stressed nutrition with high magnesium and mineral diets as an important factor in health maintenance. After all, we use the term dietary supplement and it must be understood that supplements are not to be confused as alternatives to a healthy balanced diet. The word *"supplement"* implies extra nutrient ingredients to provide health benefits over and above a balanced diet. This is the true meaning of the term *"nutraceutical,"* where nutrients are given in quantities that have biological effects that may exceed those that result from minimum or marginal intake of nutrients.

The human body is capable of absorbing about 800 milligrams of calcium each day. Unfortunately, calcium is one of the hardest minerals for the body to absorb. Many of the calcium supplements are only in the 2 to 3% absorption range, while the so-called *"great"* supplements are about only 15%. The cultures like the Hunzas, who consume over 100,000 mg of calcium each day, obviously get their 800 mg absorption, while harmlessly passing the rest in their urine and excretion. With the Okinawans, on the other hand, because of the microbes in the coral, the absorption approaches nearly 100%. Therefore, taking a 250 mg antacid calcium product, which does severe harm to the elderly by wiping out their crucial stomach acid supplies, usually results in the absorption of 5 mg (2%) calcium by the body over a 20-hour period. On the other hand, there is substantial evidence that the nutrients in coral are *absorbed in less than 20 minutes* (the blood chemistry undergoes a drastic change, for the better, in less than 20 minutes). Therefore, the 250 mg of calcium in the coral results in 250 mg being absorbed by the body in less than 20 minutes, and without destroying the crucial stomach fluids. That's almost *50 times as much calcium, 50 times as fast*. No wonder the coral calcium works so well! In addition, when people have major diseases, the consumption of a triple dose of coral provides the maximum calcium absorption.

After a suitable coral calcium material harvested from the ocean floor is selected, the material is passed through a sieve and washed gently with clean water. Knowledge of this simple process dispels the marketing myths about the solubility of coral. Coral must be sterilized under some circumstances and if unclean coral is used, it is heat sterilized at temperatures of 400 degrees Centigrade. Whilst this heat sterilization is needed for land-based, fossilized coral, it is not universally necessary for marine coral, which is usually heated at much lower temperatures. There are some who believe that the microbes would be destroyed when the coral is heated for dehydration purposes. However, rod-like bacteria can survive poor conditions, such as severe drought, heat, radiation and various chemicals. They do this by forming structures called *endospores*. A single bacterium will form a small sphere-shaped or oval-shaped spore within its cytoplasm. A tough outer covering protects this endospore. It remains dormant until favorable conditions reappear, when the spores develop into bacteria cells.

Some people have not been honest about the production processes for coral calcium, largely as a consequence of their desire to maximize economic opportunities. These people are usually using the inexpensive, low-grade coral calcium. For these reasons, I have committed the use of my likeness only in association with the premium types of coral products.

Characteristics of Marine Coral

Coral calcium is used by millions of people in both Eastern and Western societies for health benefits, but there has been a failure to consistently recognize the importance of marine versus fossilized coral. A major component of marine coral are calcium and magnesium compounds, both inorganic and organic, counting for 98% of the total product. Marine coral is tasteless and odorless. When added to water the minerals from marine coral will diffuse (mix) into water over a period of time (not immediately). Natural coral calcium can adjust the acidity and alkalinity of water over a period of time and it can assist in the removal of residual chlorine and other impurities in water. About 1% of the coral will dissolve in water within 1 hour, such as what occurs with tea bag coral, whereas 99.9% dissolves in the human stomach within minutes, such as what happens with coral capsules. In addition, coral calcium of marine origin has been shown to control bacterial contents of water.

It is important to understand that a general certificate of analysis of coral calcium should read with a calcium content of 20 to 28% (Note: the marine coral in this chapter was analyzed at 24,000 ppm or 24%) and a magnesium content of 10 to 14% (Note: the marine coral in this chapter was analyzed at 11,400 ppm or 11.4%). Lead, arsenic, mercury, cadmium and bacteria should be below critical levels. There are several common ocean pollutants in the Far East and whilst the waters surrounding Okinawa and its adjacent islands are clean and generally uncontaminated. Coral calcium must be checked for its content of PCB (Polychlorinated Biphenyls). It should be noted that the marine coral calcium, analyzed by certified laboratories in this chapter tested *"negative"* for PCB's. It is recognized that PCB is a cause of serious disease included cancer and any consumed coral calcium must be free of this environmental, man-made toxin.

On Coral Treated Water

There is no doubt that exposure of water to coral calcium results in physical and chemical changes in the water that are beneficial to health. Coral calcium causes the water to become more alkaline (shifting pH higher) and it alters the oxidation-reduction potential of water. Also, exposing coral calcium to water releases marine microbes into the water. All are considered to be advantageous for good health.

If coral tea bags cause a rapid alkalizing change to the water, the results must be treated with suspicion (probable marketing gimmick) as the coral itself can only cause the water to alkalize moderately.

Coral Trim Energized Water: Homeopathy

I wish to emphasize that I am not dismissing the use of water made with coral "tea bags," as I personally use them every day. Coral calcium exposed to water. Although only a small amount of the contained minerals dissolve in the water (about 2% whereas coral taken by the capsules result in 99%

being ionized and ready for absorption by the intestine), large amounts of biologically enhancing marine microbes are released. Because of the dramatic results to health experienced by those using the tea bag coral, there are some who make claim of a "homeopathic treatment agent." Homeopathy is the theory that disease is cured by remedies, which produce on a healthy person, effects similar to the symptoms of the diseased person (Dr. Samuel Hahnemann), the remedies being administered in minute doses. Well to begin with, that is descriptive of vitamins, which also work to cure with minute doses. Scientists are finding that this is also true with other metal nutrients, found in the coral. It is therefore logical to assume that "homeopathy" is just another term for "unknown natural nutrient," which is highly descriptive of "coral calcium."

CHAPTER 5

An Overview of Mineral and Elements Effects

The Mineral/Element Vigilantes

Minerals and trace elements work like *"vigilantes."* They can aggregate together and cooperate in supporting important body structures and function or they can oppose each other in their effects on the body. For example, calcium, magnesium, phosphorus and boron use the power of vitamin D to facilitate bone growth, development and metabolism.

Some nutritional factors change the need for trace elements. In some cases a deficiency of a vitamin may increase the need for a trace element. A good example is vitamin D deficiency resulting in the need for an increased amount of boron.

Mineral *"vigilantes"* can function alone and change their purpose or allegiance. This happens when too much of one element becomes available. Whilst boron is essential for bone growth, particularly when magnesium levels are low, too much boron is toxic. If more than 100mg of boron is taken on a daily basis, severe gastrointestinal upset, toxic central nervous system (convulsions) and even coma can occur. Of course, when the term "too much" is attached to anything, everything becomes toxic.

Trace elements and minerals function in a complex way with changing effects as a consequence of their variable concentration in body tissues and the presence of their mineral elemental companions. Thus, minerals/elements work in harmony with *"vigilante"* tendencies.

Summarizing the Biological Effects of Minerals/Elements

It is apparent that marine coral calcium is a powerhouse of mineral and elemental nutrients. There is a massive amount of literature on the effects of each micronutrient. This section summarizes the principal biological effects of each mineral/ element. The mineral/elements are discussed in alphabetical order.

Boron

Boron is found in many rocks from 10 to 200 ppm and in seawater from 4 to 6 ppm as well as in many fruits and vegetables. Avocado, kidney beans, chickpeas, peaches, beer and cider are significant sources of dietary boron. Boron is also abundant in marine organisms, especially algae at 120 ppm. Boron compounds have been known for thousands of years but the element was not discovered until 1808 by the world's best chemist at the time, Gay-Lussac This element is well absorbed and a safe daily intake is somewhere between 2 and 10 mg. Deficiency of boron leads to thinning of bones (osteoporosis), especially when combined with magnesium deficiency.

Boron seems to help prevent the formation of common types of stones in the urinary tract and it plays a role in the maintenance of healthy joints and mental alertness. A less well-known action of boron is to increase the level of male-type, sex hormones. Toxic effects of boron, as is the case for most all other elements, can be quite serious if it is taken in gram amounts. Therefore, boric acid (borax), for example, must not be taken internally because of its toxicity.

Calcium

Calcium, which makes up 3.4% of the Earth's lithosphere, and 1.6% of the human body with 100 ppm in the blood, has been discussed in much detail in this book. Vitamin D is necessary for its absorption and sunlight causes vitamin D synthesis in the body. This is why moderate exposure to sunlight is healthy. Calcium is essential for healthy bones and teeth, it facilitates muscle contraction and it is absolutely necessary for normal heart and nervous system function. In addition, calcium plays a role in blood pressure regulation, blood clotting and cancer prevention. In brief, a deficiency of calcium leads to nervous system, bone and teeth disorders and high blood pressure, especially preclampsia of pregnancy (serious high blood pressure), as well as potentially dozens of other degenerative diseases. Calcium also plays two crucial biological roles: first DNA will only replicate on a substrate of calcium thereby being crucial to biological recovery and aging, and second, calcium suppresses acid buildup thereby maintaining an alkali environment necessary to maintain oxygen. (*The Calcium Factor*, Robert R. Barefoot and Carl Reich M.D.).

Excessive calcium intake may tend to cause constipation. This effect is not usually present when marine coral calcium is taken because the balance of magnesium which may loosen the bowel off sets any constipating effects that are best avoided in people with poor kidney function and some people with urinary tract stones, especially in circumstances of dehydration.

Cesium

Cesium is found in rocks at 1 to 5 ppm, 0.07 ppm in plants and 0.06 ppm in animals (mostly in the muscle). Cesium is Mother Nature's most alkaline mineral. It is found naturally in the waters along with its cousin rubidium, of cultures such as the Hunzas in Pakistan, and the Hopi Indians in Arizona who have virtually no cancer. As a result, it has been used as a high pH cancer therapy.

Chromium

Chromium is a part of a molecule that has been called glucose tolerance factor which promotes normal fat and glucose handling by the body. Deficiencies of chromium may cause high blood cholesterol levels and intolerance to glucose (a diabetic state). It is believed that marginal chromium deficiency could be a cause of heart disease and contribute to diabetes mellitus.

Cobalt

Cobalt is part of the molecule of vitamin B12, cyanocobalamin, essential to humans in blood formation. As such it plays an indirect role in the production of DNA, the effective production of red blood cells and the efficient actions of the nervous system. It has been stated that there is no use for cobalt supplements, but, since cobalt is crucial to human survival, an intake of at least 1 mcg per day is recommended.

Copper

Copper intake is essential for normal immune function, healthy bones, joints, skin and blood vessels and it acts as an antioxidant. Deficiency of copper may result in anemia, suppressed immunity, problems with the function of nerve cells and it contributes to heart disease. The average adult contains about 100 milligrams of copper, mostly in the brain, liver, heart and kidneys. A safe intake is up to 3 mg per day and it interacts with zinc to exert its valuable functions. One common problem due to lack of copper is loss of taste sensation. Loss of taste can promote poor eating habits.

Fluoride

A deficiency of fluoride has been associated with tooth decay. Bones are made from fluoroapatite. Fluoride is added to drinking water for this reason, but some nutritionists have alleged that this is unhealthy, even though the cavity rates are practically wiped out. Excessive fluoride, especially from toothpaste products which some children eat like candy, causes skin rashes, bone problems and mottling or discoloration of teeth. Although fluoride is not classified as *"essential,"* it is essential for the production of strong bones and is considered beneficial when used in an appropriate manner.

Gold

When gold is present in the soil, which is usually the case, it accumulates in the plant's protein and chlorophyll. The roots of plants can even break up rock, liberating the gold for uptake by the plants. When animals eat the plants, gold accumulates in the proteinaceous substances, such as hair, liver, brains and muscle. Man not only eats the bread made from the golden wheat, he also eats the animals that ate the gold. In many countries, gold leaf is popular in the diet. Gold is found in man's liver, brain and muscle and human blood has been measured at 0.8 parts per billion, and 43 parts per billion have been found in human hair. Human feces and urine have been known to contain startling amounts of gold: the ash of human excretion has been known to contain one-third of an ounce per ton or over 10,000 parts per billion. The fact that gold exists in the human body in such significant amounts means that is must serve a useful function. Gold has been used successfully in some cancer treatments. Gold suspended in gel has also been used to treat wounds, resulting in rapid recovery and minimized scarring. There are hundreds of industrial processes where gold is used as a catalyst, and one day man is certain to discover that gold serves as a crucial biological catalyst in the human body.

Iodine

Iodine is an important component of thyroid hormones and it is necessary for normal growth and general body metabolism. A deficiency of iodine can cause cretinism (growth and mental retardation), low thyroid function and it has been associated with fibrocystic disease of the breasts goiter and hypothyroidism. Iodine is abundant in marine life and good dietary sources are seafood (mackerel, mussels, cod fish, prawns, etc.).

Iron

Next to calcium, iron is the most abundant mineral in the human body, crucial for maintaining oxygen. Iron permits effective oxygen transport and storage in muscles and the blood. It is the central component of hemoglobin in the red blood cells. Iron deficiency causes anemia and abnormal fat metabolism. Iron competes with other elements for absorption into the body (competition with magnesium, copper, calcium and zinc). Vitamin C enhances iron absorption and classic consequences of iron deficiency are weakness, fatigue, poor immune function and anemia. The common belief is that *"too much iron can be toxic."* The problem with this is that the words *"too much"* have never been defined. Also, United Nations Health Agency, UNESCO says that the majority of American women are anemic, as a result of iron deficiency. Although the RDA for iron is *18 mg/day* of iron, many nutritionists advocate at least *40 mg/day*. The full-term infant requires 160 mg, and the premature 240 mg during the first year of life. The 240 mg at the average 5% absorption equals 4,800 mg/year or 13 mg/day for the first year of life. The RDA for an adult is 18 mg/day. Also, for pregnant women, there is a requirement of 1 mg/day in menstruating females. At 5 mg/day this is 20 mg/day consumption. Pregnancy also increases demand for iron. Expansion of the mother's red blood cell mass requires 400 mg of iron, and the fetus and placenta require an additional 400 mg iron. Blood loss at delivery, including blood loss in the placenta, accounts for another 300 mg iron. The total requirement for a pregnancy, therefore requires about 1100 mg iron. At 5% iron absorption, this works out to *90 mg/day* requirement for a pregnant woman, but the RDA for an adult is only 18 mg/day. Thus, most women in America are beingpoisoned by *iron deficiency*.

Lithium

Lithium is found in rocks at 20 to 66 ppm, seawater at 0.18 ppm and sea animals at 1.0 ppm. Lithium is an important modulator in the conversion of essential fatty acids to postaglandins that play an important role in a variety of body functions, such as the production of white cells and T-suppressor cells. It is found in the semen, female

97

reproductive organs and the nervous system. It has been used therapeutically to treat mental disorders such as manic depression, as lithium stabilizes serotonin neurotransmissions.

Magnesium

Only about one half of the magnesium taken in the diet is absorbed into the body. Magnesium is very important in energy production, body chemistry involving protein and carbohydrate, the production of DNA and RNA and it promotes healthy structure and function of bones, the heart, muscles and blood vessels. A deficiency of magnesium may cause tiredness, mental disorders and cardiovascular disease. In fact, a marginal deficiency of magnesium has been associated with hypertension, diabetes, heart problems, migraine, PMS, osteoporosis and urinary stones. The ideal way of taking magnesium is in a ratio of two times calcium to magnesium. Magnesium occurs in this ratio in coral calcium (two parts calcium to one part magnesium). Excessive magnesium intake is best avoided in people with significant reductions in kidney or heart function.

Manganese

Manganese permits healthy function of the heart and nervous system. It plays a special role in energy production in the body, building protein and bone formation. Manganese is very important in antioxidant functions in the body because it is necessary for the function of superoxide dismutase. The results of manganese deficiency are poorly understood, but marginal deficiency of this trace element may play a role in osteoporosis and diabetes mellitus.

Molybdenum

Molybdenum is necessary for the normal handling of carbohydrates by the body. It helps in the elimination of waste products from the body, especially those resulting from protein breakdown. It is stated that molybdenum deficiency is rare but this element is often depleted from soil. Overt molybdenum deficiency causes abnormal heartbeats, migraines, anemia, partial blindness, gastrointestinal upset and mental disorders. I suspect that marginal deficiency of molybdenum occurs commonly and it may be much more important than hither to supposed.

Nickel

Nickel is found in surprisingly high concentrations in the genetic material of the body (associated with RNA and DNA). Deficiency of nickel has been reported to cause liver problems, abnormalities of reproductive function, skin rashes and decreased growth in animals. Low levels of nickel are found in kidney disease and advanced liver disease, but deficiencies are not well desorbed in humans. It appears that nickel is necessary for the normal function of several hormones and it is a co-factor for several enzymes. Nickel plays a significant role in maintaining the integrity of the cell membrane, and is heavily involved in protein replication. Nickel sensitivity can occur when it is present in jewelry. I believe that nickel may be essential in small amounts.

Potassium/Sodium/Chloride

Potassium, like sodium and chloride, is a classic *"electrolyte"* in the body. The word "electrolyte" refers to their ability to conduct electricity when dissolved in water.

Electrolytes maintain water balance in the body, play a role in muscle contractions, assist in the normal acid-alkali balance in the body and they cause the transmission of nerve impulses. In brief, potassium deficiency is associated with high blood pressure and poor heart function. Sodium excess causes high blood pressure in some people. The potassium/sodium ratio is critical for regulating the heartbeat. When the potassium level rises the heartbeat slows down. Criminals being executed are injected with potassium salt to stop their hearts from beating. Chloride is necessary for balancing pH in the body. It is also necessary for the production of stomach acid, hydrochloric acid. Deficiency leads to excessive alkalosis (high blood pH). The actions of electrolytes can be summarized as:

- Maintaining water balance
- Allowing normal muscle contraction
- Balancing acids and alkali (pH)
- Playing a role in energy production
- Producing digestive secretions
- Permitting nerve impulse transmissions

Phosphorus

Phosphorus must be present in the diet for proper balance of body chemistry, bone structure and energy production. Phosphorus joins with fats (lipids) to create phospholipids, which are vital to the function of cell membranes and to the structure of the nervous system. A deficiency of phosphorus may cause weakness, loss of appetite, central nervous system disorders and symptoms of arthritis. It is important to recognize that high levels of phosphorus intake (dietary phosphates) counteract calcium and may cause calcium deficiency.

Selenium

Selenium is essential for healthy heart and immune system function. It promotes the production of many hormones and it is necessary for the function of the important antioxidant enzyme called glutathione peroxidase. It is now recognized that selenium deficiency is common in many soils. A deficiency of selenium in the diet has been associated with cancer, heart disease, birth defects, arthritis, cataracts and autoimmune disease. Selenium toxicity can cause hair loss, fatigue and central nervous system damage. Selenium acts as an antioxidant and it works most efficiently in the presence of vitamin E.

Silicon

Silicon plays a role in cartilage formation in joints, active growth of bones and it seems to maintain the flexibility of the walls of blood vessels. In fact, low levels of silicon in animals has been associated with the development of atherosclerosis (hardening of the arteries). Silicon may be best known for its ability to support the growth of hair, nails and healthy skin. It is regarded as a safe element.

Sulfur

Sulfur is present in tissues that have a large concentration of protein e.g. connective tissues (collagen), muscles and skin. Sulfur deficiency diseases are not described per se and much of the intake of sulfur in the diet is in the form of protein. There are many actions of sulfur, but this element receives little consideration in classic nutrition. For example sulfur is necessary for normal digestion, it is a component of thiamin and biotin (B-vitamins) and it plays essential roles in body chemistry, especially oxygen utilization by cells.

Vanadium

Vanadium is an element that helps the function of the enzymes that control blood sugar. It plays a part in hormone production, bone and tooth development and reproductive function. Although vanadium deficiency is not described in humans, I believe that deficiency of this element may cause health problems. There are no classic recommendations for healthy intakes of vanadium, which is only needed in small amounts up to 100mcg per day.

Zinc

Zinc is a master metal that involves itself in hundreds of enzyme reactions in the body. Zinc is responsible for:

- Energy production in the body
- Hormone production and function
- Healthy immune function, especially of the thymus
- Normal growth and development
- Efficient detoxification in the body
- Healthy reproductive function

Whilst large amounts of zinc intake in the diet impair copper absorption, this situation is uncommon. Vitamin A can function efficiently when zinc is present. The beneficial effects of zinc are well described in the following circumstances:

- Certain types of immune deficiency
- To prevent common colds

- To help heal the skin
- To combat arthritis
- To help allay macular degeneration
- To support prostate structure and function
- To benefit several digestive diseases
- To correct some types of infertility

Overall, zinc is a very important metal nutrient.

CHAPTER 6

Minerals and Aging

Life's Journey

There are many different medical, social, behavioral and cultural attitudes to aging. Views of aging are changing as people live longer. There is no tenable definition of old age. Certainly, the distinction between chronological aging and physical aging is well recognized as *"young people"* are identified in *"aged bodies"* and octagenerians (men and women in their eighties) emerge with vitality. The arbitrary choice for the definition of *"senior years"* is 65 years, but some practitioners of geriatric medicine have demanded that their specialty services such be applied after the age of fifty years. Clearly, as we live longer, the debate about what is old or what is young will continue, especially since in the 1850's the average life expectancy was 42 years old, and at that age, everyone considered themselves to be very biologically old, and at the beginning of the 20th century the life expectancy was only 49 years. It is also interesting to note that the Bible, Genesis 6:3 states, *"Man shall not be immortal but man shall live to be 120."* Of further interest is the fact that there are locations in the world where several reach the age of 120 years old. Of final note, the Biblical patriarchs lived to over 900 years old. Thus, we know that the human body has lived for over 900 years and can, and does live today in many cultures for 120 years.

Perhaps the best way to look at aging from a medical perspective is childhood (including the young-young and young), adult life (where *"young"* or *"old"* adults exist) and the elderly or young/old, old and old/old or elite elderly. Many people would like to achieve the category of *"elite old"* which includes centenarians (elite elderly). However, the quest is for health with age. This is the real concept of *"longevity."*

The baby boomer generation that emerged after the second world war have tended to dismiss aging somewhat. The mature adult (50 years +) is beginning to see aging as a process of *"getting on with life's journey."* This attitude has both advantages and limitations; but it is close the self-actualization *"model of aging"* which is regarded by many health experts as the most appropriate view of aging.

Rhetoric and Definitions of Aging

Many definitions of aging include comments about negative physical changes, which are considered to be irreversible or culminate in death. These definitions tend to detract from the perception of aging as a dynamic process. Aging cannot be viewed in static terms. One does not go to bed young and wake up the next day with the label of being old!

The issue of overriding importance is that senior years are a payback time for earlier adverse lifestyle. It is difficult to get young people to adopt lifestyle habits as an investment for old age. However, rhetoric and definitions of old age point to preceding lifestyle as a determinant of longevity. Lifestyle has domains, e.g. nutrition, psychological well-being, substance use and abuse etc. Of all domains nutrition seems to be an under-explored area for anti-aging interventions, even though science supports this approach.

A good working definition of aging is found in the work of Dr. Erich Fromm (From *Man for Himself* Holt, Rinehart Winston Publishers, 1975). Fromm states: *"Birth is only one particular step in a continuum which begins with conception and ends with death. All that is between these two poles is a process of giving birth to one's potentialities, of bringing to life all that is potentially given in the two cells. The development of the self is never completed; even under best conditions only part of man's potentialities is realized. Man always dies before he is fully born."*

Views of Aging

The following quotations are reflections on growing old that help complete our cultural perceptions of aging in Western society.

- *"When you're forty, half of you belongs to the past – and when you are seventy, nearly all of you."* Jean Anouilh, *Time Remembered* (1939), 2.2, Tr. Patricia Moyes
- *"Age has a good mind and sorry shanks."* Pietro Aretino, *Letter to Bernardo Tasso,* 1537, Tr. Samuel Putnam
- *"To me, old age is always fifteen years older than I am."* Bernard Baruch, *News Reports,* Aug. 20, 1955
- *"Years steal/ Fire from the mind as vigour from the limb;/ And Life's enchanted cup but sparkles near the brim."* Byron, *Childe Harold's Pilgrimage* (1812- 18), 3.8
- *"We must not take the faults of our youth into our old age, for old age brings with it its own defects."* Goethe, Quoted in Johann Peter Eckermann's *Conversations with Goethe,* August 16, 1824

- *"Few people know how to be old."* La Rochefoucauld, *Maxims* (1665), Tr. Kenneth Pratt
- *"Growing old is no more than a bad habit which a busy man has no time to form."* Andre Maurois, quoted in *The Aging American* (1961)
- *"Ask who wants to live to be a hundred, and the answer is the person who is ninety-nine."* Betty Comden, *Break the Other Leg* (1994)
- *"The man who has lived the longest is not he who has spent the greatest number of years, but he who has had the greatest sensibility of life."* Rousseau, Emile (1762)
- *"Every man desires to live long, but no man would be old."* Jonathan Swift, *Thoughts on Various Subjects* (1711)
- *"They live ill who expect to live always."* Publilius Syrus, *Moral Sayings* (1st C.B.C.), 457, Tr. Darius Lyman

Addressing Theories of Aging

There are several distinct pathways to aging, which are classified under the terms biological, sociological and psychological. These pathways operate together in the aging process, but within the context of this book I wish to examine focused aspects of nutritional support, especially mineral intake, and interpret its importance in relationship to theories of aging. I stress that aging is a multi-factorial issue, but there is evidence that mineral intake seems to be an important common denominator for longevity. The functions of minerals and elements "touch" every theory of aging in a logical manner and form a common thread of understanding of the aging process.

Table 8 summarizes several theories of aging. We know that aging is not completely understood and this is evidenced by the number of hypothesis that exist to explain the phenomenon. I stress that no single theory of aging, is all encompassing, but nutrition and the biological function of minerals provides a core understanding (Table 8).

Table 8
Seven Theories of Aging. Whilst Many Complex Factors Operate, Minerals and Elements Play a Pivotal Role in all of These Proposed Mechanisms of Aging

THEORY OF AGING	COMMENT
1. Free radical theories	Free radicals (reactive oxygen species) cause oxidative damage. Antioxidants of many types occur in the body or in nature and they often require essential elements to function e.g. selenium, zinc.
2. Cross-link theories	Chemical links occur in collagen and other tissues. The basis of this process is aberrant mineral calcium deposition. Balances between and biological cross linkers e.g. copper and magnesium are very important.
3. Immunologic theories	Autoimmunity increases with age. The thymus shrinks. Many factors involved but metal- dependent enzyme systems support immune function and specific metals are obligatory for immune functions e.g. zinc.

4. Mutation and Error Theories	Mistakes in DNA replication or RNA function result in aging or age-related disease e.g. cancer. Enzyme functions and chemical processes are all mineral related.
5. Aging Programs	A program may exist in the gene for a specific number of all diversions. Again minerals would operate.
6. Stress Theories	Stress is cumulative and lifestyle related, nutritional and mineral deficiencies enhance stress.
7. Repair Budget Theories	Environmental and lifestyle issues alter the investment of an organism in tissue repair. Tissue repair is dependent on nutrition, especially mineral support.

Of all theories of aging the free radical theory has gained most interest in contemporary medical research. Free radicals are parts of chemical compounds that are highly reactive with tissues. They are positively charged and therefore thrive in an acidic body environment that is the result of deficiencies in minerals, especially calcium. Oxygen is capable of reacting with tissues, resulting in free radical generation. The body produces many compounds to *"mop up free radicals"* but among the most important free radical generators or *"quenchers"* are metals. For example, excessive iron can generate free radical damage, whereas zinc and selenium support body systems that *"quench"* free radicals. In this circumstance, these elements are antioxidants with actions similar to vitamin E, coenzyme Q10, green tea, soyisoflavones, etc.

Many scientists believe that the repeated exposure of the body to free radicals, which thrive in a mineral-deficient acidic environment, is a fundamental process in aging. Many studies now confirm that adopting a diet high in antioxidants, like the diet of Okinawans, is an important issue in the promotion of healthy aging.

Longevity: "The Nitty-Gritty"

Humankind today has the demonstrated potential to live one hundred years, but to understand the way to achieve this goal is to examine the main reasons that account for premature death. Most people will live into the seventh decade, but then the common killer diseases often take hold. These frequent killers are heart disease, cancer and the consequences of several common chronic diseases. If heart disease and other cardiovascular disorders such as hypertension and stroke could be eliminated it is estimated that up to two decades could be added to the current average lifespan of seventy years. To prevent cancer may add another five to ten years. Thus, addressing these common killer diseases would help humankind achieve the centenarian goal.

Minerals and Healthy Heart

The eradication of coronary heart disease is a major public health initiative for this millennium. Carl Reich M.D. has pointed to lifestyle issues and several natural interventions as a logical way to cardiovascular health. When Dr. Reich died a few years ago, the local newspapers hailed him as a "Man Before His Time" and "The Father of Preventive Medicine." Of particular interest is the pivotal role that elements and minerals play in cardiovascular health. Magnesium is necessary for energy production in every cell. In addition, it has an important job of balancing the physiological activity of potassium and calcium in the body. There is evidence that magnesium can help the heart withstand heart attack, and some studies have shown that magnesium, if given at the time of the initial cardiac event, results in a reduced death rate several weeks after the event. Scandinavian and Israeli studies showed the beneficial outcome of administering magnesium during heart attacks in double-blind, controlled clinical studies.

Magnesium may have a role in normalizing blood lipid levels, and animal studies have shown that supplementing the diet with magnesium can assist in reducing the severity of atherosclerosis. A most important feature of magnesium is its role in maintaining normal heart rhythm. Magnesium deficiencies are associated with cardiac arrhythmias, which are life-threatening situations. However, excessive magnesium can also alter heart function, so the amount used is critical. Magnesium supplementation has also shown some benefit for patients with peripheral vascular disease and in patients with congestive heart failure.

The RDA of magnesium is 350 mg per day for men (280 mg/day for women), and it is likely that a typical Western diet may be deficient in this material. This is especially true among people using diuretics. With the exception of an individual with kidney disease, including kidney failure, magnesium supplements are generally considered safe. However, magnesium intake must be balanced with adequate calcium intake in the diet.

Calcium is important for, among other things, regulating blood pressure (as is magnesium). It also may play a role in raising HDL and lowering LDL. Calcium, magnesium, potassium, and sodium are of critical importance, but they must be used in balanced amounts. There is an ongoing fluctuation and *"balancing act"* in the body that regulates these minerals. For this reason, supplementation with these minerals should be supervised.

The British Medical Research Council recently completed a 10-year study that looked at the health of *5,000 men* aged between 45 and 59. *Only one percent* of those who regularly drank more than one-half liter (about one-half U.S. quart) of milk a day suffered heart attacks in the study period, against *ten percent* of those who drank *no milk at all* (a *tenfold* reduction). Also, drinking more than the one-half of a liter further reduced the incidence of heart attack. Dr. Ann Fehily, one of the team of researchers, states that *"the association between milk drinking and lower heart attack risk was **absolutely clear**, and there was no significance about what type of milk: full, semi-skimmed or full-skimmed."* Thus, the essential ingredient was *calcium*.

An essential trace mineral, selenium is needed to produce **glutathione peroxidase**, a powerful antioxidant enzyme. In recent years, glutathione has been identified as one of the most important protective antioxidant agents – in this case, an enzyme. Vitamin E and selenium work synergistically, and vitamin E protects against selenium toxicity. The exact heart-protective mechanism of this mineral is not known, but epidemiologic studies show a relationship between low selenium levels and higher risk of heart disease. Selenium intake is measured in micrograms, and the RDA is 70 mcg for men and 55 mcg for women. The National Research Council states an optimal range of intake of 50 to 200 mcg. It is best to take selenium along with the other antioxidant nutrients, rather than alone.

Table 9

Summarizes the Effect of Minerals on Common Cardiovascular Disease

Calcium	Calcium can decrease total cholesterol and triglycerides; calcium deficiencies can promote atherosclerosis. Calcium eliminates the acid attacking the muscle tissue of the artery, thereby eliminating the need for the body to produce plaque to strengthen the artery, thus eliminating heart disease.
Copper	Copper deficiency is associated with high blood cholesterol and decreased HDL. Copper also provides the elasticity to prevent aneurysms.
Iron	Iron may contribute to atherom formation.
Chromium	Chromium supplements may raise HDL and lower total blood cholesterol and LDL. Deficiency of chromium is a risk factor for arteriosclerosis.
Magnesium	Magnesium deficiency is more common than recognized. It can result

	in an increased risk of coronary disease, sudden cardiac health, heart attack, and abnormal heart rhythm.
Selenium	Low blood levels of selenium predispose to atheroma.
Zinc	Atherosclerosis may reduce zinc blood levels. Zinc may exert both beneficial and untoward effects on blood lipids.

Whilst the prevention of cardiovascular disease and cancer are highly complex issues, nutritional factors such as mineral intake plays a major role in the causation and progression of these disorders. Longevity has been associated with groups of people (Hunzas, Okinawans, etc.) who eat vegetable foods that are high in nutrients and essential trace elements (see Davis 1975 and Benet 1976). I stress that mineral intake may not be the only factor, but it certainly forms a common thread of importance in the prevention and treatment of fatal diseases. It is valuable to explore how minerals and elements may operate to prevent and treat disease. The minerals that are discussed are all found in coral calcium which may contribute to longevity in Okinawans. These observations on minerals and health are more than a coincidence.

CHAPTER 7

Minerals Maintain Life: Elemental Chemistry

Minerals, Elements and Health

Nutritionists and caregivers have broadly classified elements or minerals into *"toxic"* types or *"nutrient"* types. However, minerals that are traditionally considered "toxic" may be very valuable in small doses in biological systems. For example, the toxic element arsenic has been shown in recent research to have a beneficial health role in minute traces in the diet. Although discoveries are made in biochemistry about the role of certain minerals or elements or biological processes, minerals assumed to be toxic are generally not supplemented in the diet. As knowledge increases, we may have to redefine mineral *"toxicity."* What was once considered toxic and undesirable in terms of small amounts of certain minerals may emerge as quite desirable for health. Also, every nutrient on Earth is toxic in high enough quantities. Even water can kill, and water is essential for life.

An element described as toxic is best kept as low as possible in terms of body exposure. A simple way to assist in gradual reduction of toxic mineral is to take vitamin C in amounts from 0.5 mg to 2 grams per day, or more. Table 10 lists elements that are regarded as toxic. In Appendix A the sources and consequences of toxic elements are reviewed in more complete manner.

Table 10
A List of the Principal Toxic Elements. Their
Source and Adverse Effects are Described in Appendix A

Aluminium (Al)	Mercury (Hg)
Antimony (Sb)	Nickel (Ni)
Arsenic (As)	Thallium (TI)
Cadmium (Cd)	Tin (Sn)
Lead (Pb)	Uranium (U)

Nutrient Minerals

Table 11 summarizes essential, nutrient minerals and their recommended intakes expressed as US Reference Daily Intake (RDI). The RDI is supposed to provide guidance for average levels of supplementation (or dietary content) to support essential body functions, but I believe as do many other scientists, that these RDIs are often too conservative.

Table 11
When Nutritionally Essential Elements are Low or Deficient, the US Reference Daily Intake (RDI) Levels Provide Guidance for Supplementation. The RDIs for Elements or Minerals are the Daily Intakes Recommended for Essential Body Functions

Element	RDI **
Calcium	1000 milligrams***
Chromium	120 micrograms
Copper	2 milligrams
Iodine	150 micrograms
Magnesium	400 milligrams
Manganese	2 milligrams
Selenium	70 micrograms
Zinc	15 milligrams

Many minerals are considered "essential" for body functions. The term essential implies that their absence or deficiency can lead to serious disease. However, there are a lot of minerals that appear to play an important role in vital body functions but they do not claim the label "essential" although I suspect that many are essential for health. The value of many elements and minerals for health maintenance still remains underexplored. A list of nutrient elements is given in Table 12. In Appendix B a more complete account of the source, optimum intake and consequence of imbalance is discussed.

Table 12

A List of Classic Nutrient Elements. A More Complete Account of Their Actions is Given in Appendix B

Boron (B)	Molybdenum (Mo)
Calcium (Ca)	Phosphorus (P)
Chromium (Cr)	Potassium (K)
Cobalt (Co)	Selenium (Se)
Copper (Cu)	Silicon (Si)
Iodine (I)	Sodium (Na)
Iron (Fe)	Strontium (Sr)
Lithium (Li)	Vanadium (V)
Magnesium (Mg)	Zinc (Zn)
Manganese (Mn)	

RDAs, RDIs are Often Underestimated

Several researchers point to evidence that many U.S. Recommended Daily Intakes of nutrients (RDIs) are too low. The term RDI has generally replaced the concepts of RDA. The US Reference Intakes that are recommended for vitamins and minerals has tended to focus on amounts that *"prevent"* deficiencies. Whilst deficiencies of essential nutrients are to be avoided at all costs, we know that vital nutrients are responsible for sustaining the chemistry of life and many are required in abundance. In addition, there is a clear difference between an amount of vitamins and minerals just to *"get by"* without deficiency diseases and an amount required to exert treatment benefits or insurance for optimal health. It should be noted once again, that the long-living cultures that are virtually disease-free consume over 100 times the RDA of many nutrients and suffer the side effects of perpetual health and life.

Despite this, one should not subscribe to the simple notion that more is necessarily better, but nutritionists have started to think in terms of optimal daily intake (ODI). The ODI of nutrient often involves the recommendation that higher amounts of nutrients are required than are classified under the standard RDI system. The RDI system is a series of concepts with limitations, which have never undergone scientific scrutiny. This is why in all literature the terms *"may be toxic"* and *"could be toxic"* are always used. This allows for confirmation by *"insinuation."* The fact is that *"no recognized scientific study has ever been done to confirm these concepts"* with limitations. In conclusion, many leading physicians and nutritionists have recommended levels of nutrient intake that exceed RDIs. This modern trend is in keeping with my proposal that the common denominator for health is abundant nutrient mineral and element supply. The Hunzas and Okinawans help to prove my point of view.

Placing Minerals into Perspective

The word minerals refers to their presence in the forming of the earth's crust. Minerals build rock formations and as we have discussed the coral reefs. Rocks tend to be broken down into tiny fragments that form soil as a consequence of many millions of years of exposure to changing climates. The same thing happens in the coral reef, but in the oceans living organisms assist in the breakdown of coral, which occurs from weathering. The basis of soil in mountainous, rocky areas is a high mineral content derived from rock erosions. Soil *"teams with bacteria"* that bring mineral residues into food chains for living organisms. Minerals are passed to plants which, in turn, pass them on to animals. The series of mineral conversions that occur on dry land occurs by somewhat similar mechanisms in the oceans.

To understand mineral contents of plant and animal tissues, one can study the residual as content of burned tissues. Minerals of abundance in the body include sodium, potassium, calcium, phosphorus and magnesium, but trace minerals, which are essential for life, are also present. These include small amounts of zinc, iodine, manganese, copper and even metal poisons such as arsenic. Only lead, mercury and cadmium, all of which are considered extremely toxic, are missing. It is important to recognize that metals and minerals are responsible for many metabolic processes in living tissues, especially the function of structural proteins and enzymes.

Simplifying the Characteristics of Bioelements

Let us simplify the basic physical characteristics that would be required by any bioelement, such as calcium, which has the job of participating in almost all biochemical functions. Considering calcium, it provides basic structural building material in tissues that can readily be removed and replaced. To begin with, the ideal bioelement (calcium) would have to be abundant; the most common elements in the Earth's crust are oxygen at 49%, silicon at 26%, aluminium at 7.5%, iron at 4.7%, calcium at 3.4%, magnesium at 1.9%, hydrogen at 0.88%, titanium at 0.55%, phosphorus at 0.12%, carbon at 0.09%, manganese at 0.08%, sulfur at 0.03%, and all others at less than these elements (see Table 13). The chemically active element calcium is appropriately found in a high range of concentration in the Earth's crust. (Calcium comprises 3.4% of the earth's crust.)

Table 13
Elemental Composition of the Earth's Crust
Versus the Human Body

Element	% Earth's Crust	% Human Body
Oxygen	49.00	65.00
Silicon	26.00	trace
Aluminium	7.50	trace
Iron	4.70	1.00
Calcium	**3.40**	**1.60**
Sodium	2.60	0.30
Potassium	2.40	0.40
Magnesium	1.90	0.05
Hydrogen	0.88	10.00
Titanium	0.55	trace
Chlorine	0.19	0.30
Phosphorus	0.12	0.90
Carbon	0.09	18.00
Manganese	0.08	0.00
Sulfur	0.03	0.25
TOTAL	**99.46**	**100.00**

Note: All other non-man-made elements (77 elements) make up 0.54% of the Earths crust.

It should be noted that all of the elements listed in Table 13 can be found in the human body, and the one that is lowest in concentration in the Earth's crust, carbon, is the basic building block element of life as we know it. However, it is basically only a *"structural"* component, and must be chemically compounded with the element hydrogen in molecular form to be an active "functional" ingredient in the body. This compounding renders carbon less reactive, as it must always be attached to one or more hydrogen atoms, than the simple element calcium that is required for diverse biochemical activity.

Some Technical Considerations

The most abundant element, oxygen, is also never found unattached in its essential form. It has six electrons in its outer second orbital, and is very aggressive in trying to fill up this orbital with two more electrons. This trait is known as electro-negativity, and oxygen is number one in chemical *"aggressiveness."* The giving up or sharing of electrons resulting in elemental bonding, by definition, represents a chemical reaction. As a rule, elements with outer orbitals that are less than half full tend to give up these electrons, and elements with outer electron orbitals more than half full tend to acquire electrons to fill this orbital. Thus, oxygen preferentially binds itself to elements with outer orbitals not only less than half full, but also with the most available electrons.

Contenders Among the Most Active Bioelements

The list of most abundant elements with less than half full but that have the most electrons in their outer orbital for oxygen to *"grab"* are as follows: sulfur with six electrons, phosphorus with five electrons, silicon and carbon with four electrons, aluminum with three electrons, iron with three or two electrons, magnesium and calcium with two electrons, and sodium and potassium with one electron. Since the stability of the molecules formed depends on the number of electrons shared, and since oxygen is an integral part of life as we know it, we must remove the elements to which oxygen will most readily attach. Thus sulfur, phosphorus, silicon, carbon, and aluminum must be removed from the list of elements, which were contenders for the most active biochemical element.

This leaves sodium, potassium, magnesium, and calcium as the most logical contenders. It should be noted that sodium and potassium are alkali metals, and magnesium and calcium are alkaline Earth metals, or in other words, these elements all exhibit the physical property of producing alkaline solutions, pH greater than 7, when exposed to water. Thus it would be logical that most of the body fluids, in which the biochemical activity occurs with one or more of these elements, should have a pH greater than 7. However, the higher the pH of the fluids rises above 7, the more corrosive they become, and although certain restricted parts of the body, such as the stomach, can contain corrosive acidic fluids, every cell throughout the body definitely cannot.

Maintaining the Balance of Alkalinity and Acidity

Both sodium and potassium produce very caustic and corrosive solutions and must be balanced with anions, such as chlorides, to bring their pH down to approximate neutrality at pH 7. On the contrary, both calcium and magnesium produce mildly alkaline solutions with a variety of anions, and thus require less dependence on the presence of other specific ions. Although all of these last four elements will be found to be important for body functions, calcium and magnesium appear to be emerging as the most flexible.

Another trait that would be desired would be biological efficiency, or in other words the ability of an ion to attach to a larger number of nutrient polar radicals or proteins. There are a large number of polar molecules, the most common being water, and glucose. When under the influence of a strong electrical field, such as the negative cell surface mostly made up of phospholipids, the polar compounds tend to stack themselves by having their oppositely charged ends face each other, creating the stack. Since the outer end of this aligned stack is negative, the negative cell surface has thereby propagated its electrical field out to the end of the stack, where, at this point it can attach itself to a cation (positive ion). Both calcium and magnesium ions have two electrons missing from their outer orbitals which allows them to attract more of the polar stack extending out from the cell surface, thus emerging once again over sodium and potassium ions which have only just one electron missing from their outer orbitals.

Simple Theories of Electricity and Nutrient Elements

This process of electric field propagation is very common in nature and can be better understood by providing a simple illustration: dry sand readily pours out of a bucket when turned upside down; however, when a bucket of wet sand is turned upside down, the sand comes out in one whole piece, retaining its shape. This occurs because a particle of sand, like the phospholipid cell surface, is made up with oxygen on its surfaces. When wet, the polar water stacks up from all of the surfaces, thus propagating the negative fields outwardly until they meet and try to repel each other from all sides, resulting in each sand grain remaining suspended with enough force to defy gravity.

This situation is similar to the two like poles of magnetic levitation repelling each other to defy gravity, thereby allowing a train to remain suspended in mid air. With the water-suspended sand, the crystals on the edge are prevented from being pushed off the stack by the force of the water surface tension. Similarly, this electric field propagated out from the cell is a strong force in organizing the positively charged cation biochemical workhorses, such as calcium. The most common polar compounds in the extracellular cell fluid are water and glucose. Sodium, potassium, calcium and magnesium cations are all frequently affected by this electrical field propagation, with other cations less frequently affected; however; once the stack breaks from the membrane, one element, calcium, is vastly superior in assisting nutrients into the cell.

Calcium Emerges as the Key Bioelement

Another ability that the master biochemical element must have is the ability to readily release the stacked polar nutrients once they have entered the cell. Magnesium has two electrons in its outer third orbital, while calcium has two electrons in its outer fourth orbital, and also has eight electrons with ten vacancies in its inner third orbital. Thus, because of its larger size and electron vacancies, calcium's electrons are much more loosely bound than are magnesium's, thereby allowing calcium to more readily give up its electrons to proteins and to polar nutrients. For example, calcium has a greater ability than magnesium to cross link with other molecules.

Calcium can bind to seven oxygen locations on a protein while still holding onto a water molecule, while magnesium can only bind to three oxygen locations on a protein while holding on to two water molecules. The water molecules exchange at a rate five thousand times greater, and therefore much more easily, for calcium than for magnesium. Calcium is a larger ion than magnesium, therefore it moves faster. Calcium binds to the central atom of biologically important coordination compounds, ligands, both ten thousand times as fast and ten thousand times as strong as does magnesium. Since all of these abilities give calcium the most chemical flexibility to carry out the myriad of biological duties required to sustain life, *"calcium"* can rightfully claim the title of *"King of the Bioelements."*

Some Key Chemical Reactions of Calcium

Of course there are many other reasons why calcium predominates so readily over the other elements in biological importance. It has been known since the time of the Romans as a strong building material, with much of the calcium in the cement being both removable and replaceable without the structure collapsing. This is also one of the most important properties of the human body. Whilst calcium is considered to be the biological glue that keeps all of the cells in the body from coming apart, much of it can be removed or replaced without breakup of the structure.

Another important property that has been discussed in the research literature is calcium's ability to behave like an octopus and bind to several different elements at once, enabling it to bind and bunch up long proteins, an ability necessary to regulate entry of ions into the cell. Since ionization is required to produce a voltage that will regulate entrance through the cell membrane, calcium comes out the winner as, to produce a specific voltage, it requires the least of ionization. For example, 70 millivolts of potential difference between the outer and inner layer of cell membrane can be produced by the ionization of only 507 parts per million of calcium, while 933 parts per million of potassium would be required to produce the same voltage.

And last but not least, calcium also has the unique ability to form a soluble (mono) orthophosphate, which, in combination with calcium bicarbonate, acts as a crucial component of a pH buffer system that holds the extra cellular fluid in the 7.4 pH range. Also, as calcium bonds to the phosphates, it liberates sodium and potassium, allowing them to form alkaline salts, as well as combining with bicarbonates to produce mild chemical buffers such as sodium bicarbonate in the pH 7.7 range. This alkaline pH buffering mechanism is crucial in allowing glucose to break down into the four nucleotides - adenine, guanine, cytosine and thiamin – that are the basic building blocks of DNA. When the pH drops below 6.5, becoming acidic, the glucose breaks down into lactic acid, thus creating even more acidity and starving the cell of the basic building materials it requires for DNA replication.

Summarizing the Role of Calcium as the "King of Bioelements"

In summary, calcium is one of the most abundant elements on Earth. It is small enough to have the mobility to enable it to pass through small openings, yet it is large enough to have enough electrons in enough orbitals to influence a variety of bonding with other nutrient compounds. However, it has significantly less electrons in its outer orbital than most of the other common elements, thereby minimizing its entrapment with the most common element, oxygen. Calcium is the basic ingredient responsible for producing strong cellular building materials while retaining the ability to be removed and replaced without causing the collapse of the structure. Very little calcium ionization is required to produce necessary biochemical voltages. Calcium is the only element that can produce the crucial buffered pH of 7.4 required to DNA synthesis. Calcium is clearly the *"King of the Bioelements."*

CHAPTER 8

The Calcium Factor

What Calcium Does

Mention calcium and everyone thinks immediately of healthy bones and teeth. Whilst skeletal health is absolutely dependant on calcium in the diet, hundreds of thousands of scientific publications point to the role of calcium in many fundamental body functions that sustain life. The element calcium has chemical actions that are powerful, flexible, and life sustaining to the degree that it rightfully claims the title "King of Bioelements." Table 14 summarizes some of the biological roles that are adopted by calcium in body structure and function.

Table 14
Observations on the Biological Role of Calcium

FUNCTION	COMMENT
Bones and teeth	Inadequate calcium intake is associated with rickets, osteomalacia, osteoporosis and poor dentition. Bone tissue is metabolically active and releases stores of calcium to maintain blood levels, which are controlled by vitamin D. calcitonin and parathormone.

Biological cement (tissue glue)	Calcium binds several elements at once which accounts for its ability to regulate entry of ions into cells. Calcium participates in cell adhesion maintaining the integrity of the linings of body cavities and the skin.
Key regulatory ion for cells	Calcium regulates pH and the cell membranes voltage and channel openings, thereby bringing nutrients into cells.
Anti-cancer effects	Many believe in a direct cause-effect relationship between calcium deficiency and cancer It is required for normal DNA function. It protects against mutations and tends to produce tissue alkalinity, which inhibits the spread of cancer.
Nervous system	Essential for nerve impulse conduction.
Cardiovascular health	Calcium ions are required for cardiac contraction. Calcium may lower blood pressure. And it tends to reduce blood lipids.
Muscle function	Required for skeletal muscle contraction.
Allergy/immunity	Calcium is a second messenger in cells for example when signals are given to cells of the immune system, calcium transmits the signal into action inside the cells.

Unified health concept	Calcium has so many actions in biological systems that it's balanced supply is required for almost all major body functions.
Miscellaneous	Essential for cell division, immune function, enzyme activity and hormone production.

Many Health Benefits of Calcium

There are several recognized benefits of calcium supplementation other than their obvious effects in the maintenance of healthy skeletal function. Many studies have addressed the possible role of calcium intake in the prevention or amelioration of bone loss, cancer of the colon, hypertension, and preclampsia of pregnancy (NIH Consensus on Osteoporosis, 1984). Calcium has been demonstrated to have a mild antihypertensive effect. In a double-blind crossover study, 48 subjects with moderate hypertension received 1g/day of calcium or a placebo for eight weeks. Reductions in blood pressure were noted in the subjects during calcium administration. In addition, reductions in blood lipids (cholesterol and triglycerides) have been observed in long-term studies, thereby giving calcium a clear role in the promotion of cardiovascular wellness.

Of prevailing theories of the pathogenesis (causation) of osteoporosis, dietary calcium deficiency gains widespread support. However, other factors, such as estrogen deficiency, lack of exercise, vitamin and trace element deficiency, pollution, and a variety of lifestyle factors may play a role. Scientists have coined the term "type III" osteoporosis. There are many reviews of the association of osteoporosis with a variety of conventional medical therapies, including corticosteroids, anticoagulants, diuretics, anticonvulsants, certain psychoactive medications, and excessive smoking and drinking of alcohol. The association of osteoporosis with a variety of other disorders or diseases is well recognized. Such conditions include diabetes mellitus, thyroid disease, chronic airways (lungs) disease, and arthritis of multiple causes. The association of osteoporosis with osteoarthritis is particularly strong. They often go *"hand in hand."*

Diet and Osteoporosis

Allan Gaby M.D. has drawn particular attention to diet as a determinant of bone and joint health. In several clinical series, approximately one-half of all groups of male chronic alcoholics may have osteoporosis. Other dietary factors that have been associated with the development of osteoporosis include excessive protein intake in the diet (Table 15), excessive phosphorus consumption, and high sodium intake. Some studies indicate that individuals who maintain a vegetarian diet may have less osteoporosis than omnivorous individuals, but the data is conflicting.

Table 15 emphasizes the relatively strong relationship between animal protein intake and hip fractures. The occurrence of hip fractures can be largely attributed to osteoporosis. The type of protein in the diet (animal versus vegetable) seems important, with vegetable protein affording a preventive effect. The whole issue of food processing as a cause of reductions in the nutrient value of many foods has been well reviewed, and food processing is believed to contribute indirectly to the causation of osteoporosis and other chronic diseases that may be related to nutrient deficiency. Food grown in mineral depleted soils is believed to play a role in promoting osteoporosis as a consequence of calcium and trace metal deficiency.

Osteoporosis:
Increasing and Devastating

There are some interesting observations on a possible temporal (overtime) increase in the prevalence of osteoporosis. Studies performed in England and Sweden show evidence of a rise in the documented number of osteoporotic-related fractures over an approximate 30 to 40- year period from the 1950s to the 1980s. The reasons for this occurrence are not clear, but they could be diet related. It is well recognized that the occurrence of hip fractures in the elderly is often a major milestone in life because it may often signal placement of the elderly in chronic nursing care facilities. Many of the victims of hip fracture never recover ambulant functions, even after surgical therapy. Hip fracture is a major public health concern in the elderly for which preventive strategies to reduce osteoporosis and enhance safety should be instituted.

Table 15
Relationship Between Animal Protein Intake
and Hip Fracture Rate

Country	Animal protein intake (approximate g/day)	Hip fracture rate (per 100,000 people)
South Africa-Blacks	10.4	6.8
New Guinea	16.4	3.1
Singapore	24.7	21.6
Yugoslavia	27.3	27.6

Hong Kong	34.6	45.6
Israel	42.5	93.2
Spain	47.6	42.4
Holland	54.3	87.7
United Kingdom	56.6	118.2
Denmark	58.0	165.3
Sweden	59.4	187.8
Finland	60.5	111.2
Ireland	61.4	76.0
Norway	66.6	190.4
United States	72.0	144.9
New Zealand	77.8	119.0

Note: These countries also establish the trend that hip fractures are less due to proximity to the equator, or the exposure to sun.

Several studies show that women experience a loss of bone density when they have a daily calcium consumption of less than approximately 400 mg/day. Loss of bone density is much less in those women who have a prolonged calcium intake of approximately 750 mg/day. Although some studies have failed to show a major beneficial effect of calcium supplementation in preventing or reversing osteoporosis, an overwhelming body of opinion is in favor of calcium supplementation as a preventive measure for osteoporosis.

Accepting the importance of dietary calcium supplementation, the amount and chemical type of calcium and the source and format of calcium in the diet are believed to be important variables. The Recommended Daily Allowance (RDA) for calcium in the diet is variable (on average 1,000 mg/day) for adults and 1,000 to 2,000 mg/day for young adults or postmenopausal women. I believe that these are underestimates. Several studies have indicated that calcium intake in many diets may often be below the RDA, especially in the elderly. There are a number of adverse effects of taking too much calcium in the diet, but this usually occurs if the individual is otherwise not healthy, and usually occurs when the individual had little exposure to sunshine resulting in a drop in the production of the calcium regulators calcitonon and inositol triphosphate. Caution is suggested with the administration of calcium (and magnesium) supplements in the presence of renal failure, but reports of interference of excessive dietary calcium intake with zinc assimilation are probably not of clinical significance.

Calcium: Bones and Teeth

Skeletal health and dental health go hand in hand. Calcium is an important factor for the promotion of healthy teeth, and administration of calcium in a dose of 1 g/day for six months has been observed to have beneficial effects in periodontal disease. In these studies, bone growth is noted as a consequence of calcium administration in some individuals at sites where alveolar bone loss had occurred. Overall, clinical investigations show that calcium supplementation appears to reduce tooth mobility (loosening) and bleeding gums, with coincidental improvement in gingival inflammation. There is a very clear link between periodontal disease (disease of teeth and gums) and general health. The relationship between poor dental health and cardiovascular disease is particularly strong. Since cardiovascular disease is the number one killer in Western society, the interest benefits of calcium on oral health are particularly important for longevity.

Diseases and Oral Health

Thirty years ago, Professor Samuel C. Miller, D.D.S., of the New York School of Dentistry proposed a relationship between poor dental hygiene and many different diseases. His work was ignored for a decade until these relationships were further examined. In particular, there seems to be a close link between a variety of cardiovascular diseases and dental health.

Several studies reported in the medical literature indicate the possibility of bacterial translocation (migration and travel) to the bloodstream. Bacteria that are found in the mouth can collect in atheromatous plaques (cholesterol deposits) that are found in arteries throughout the body. Organisms that have been identified as having this translocation potential include *Helicobacter pylori* (associated with gastritis and peptic ulcer) and *Chlamydia pneumoniae* (a common cause of lung infection).

In animal experiments performed at the University of Minnesota, dental researchers showed that bacteria from dental plaque were able to escape into the bloodstream and produce small blood clots. In these experiments, large amounts of certain bacteria (*Streptococcus sanguis and Porphyromonas gingivalis* — common oral inhabitants) caused irregular heartbeats and early signs of a heart attack. It appears that these common bacteria that are present in the mouth have clotting factors on their surface that cause blood to coagulate (especially *Streptococcus sanguis*).

Scientific studies at the University of Toronto, Canada,

have shown the presence of immune markers from oral bacteria in cholesterol-containing plaques (atherosclerosis) – suggesting but not proving a relationship between oral bacteria and atherosclerosis. These findings are supported by population studies from the National Institutes of Health and the State University that links the presence of gum disease with the occurrence of cardiovascular disease, coronary heart disease, and stroke.

The associations of poor dental hygiene and heart disease have been extended to lung disease and peptic ulcer disease. Overall, it seems that dental health is a much more important determinant of general health than medicine has previously recognized.

Calcium and Cancer

The role of dietary calcium or calcium supplements in the prevention of cancer is attracting increasing interest. Epidemiological observations show an inverse correlation between dietary calcium intake and the risk of developing colon cancer. Calcium administration has been observed to reduce proliferative (growth) activity in colonic mucosa (lining of the large bowel). This proliferative activity is an important prelude to colon cancer development. The NIH Consensus Conference on Optimal Calcium Intake (1994) did not recommend that calcium intake be increased to combat colon cancer. However, apart from minor conflicting data and problems of methodological interpretation of some studies, the author believes that the NIH Consensus Conference has taken the wrong position on calcium and colon cancer and that calcium intake plays a potential role in preventing colon cancer. It should be recognized that more than 135,000 cases of colon cancer are diagnosed each year in the United States, and the American Cancer Society has stressed preventive efforts to combat this common killer disease.

Calcium and perhaps other minerals such as selenium may be important preventatives against colon cancer. Whilst most of the evidence of cancer preventive effects have focused on colon cancer, I believe that calcium may also prevent other types of gastrointestinal cancer, and breast cancer or prostate cancer.

The January 14, 1999 issue of the Phoenix Republic wrote in an article entitled *"Calcium Reduces Tumors"* that the New England Journal of Medicine reported *"adding calcium to the diet can keep you from getting tumors in your large intestine."* Then the February 1999 issue of the *Reader's Digest* wrote in an article entitled *"The 'Superstar' Nutrient"* that the Journal of the American Medical published "when the participants consumption reached *1,500 milligrams of calcium a day, cell growth in the colon improved toward normal* (this means that the cancer was reversed)". In the same article, the Digest reported, "in 1997 the large federally financed trial found that a diet containing *1,200 milligrams of calcium significantly lowered blood pressure in adults."* Then the May 3, 1999 edition of *US World News Report* wrote in an article entitled *"Calcium's Powerful Mysterious Ways,"* that *"Researchers are increasingly finding that the humble mineral calcium plays a major role in warding off major illnesses from high blood pressure to colon cancer"* and that *"You name the disease, and calcium is beginning to have a place there"* (David McCarron, a nephrologist at Oregon Health Sciences University).

Unfortunately, most doctors have not heard the news that their own journals and major newspapers and magazines are reporting that natural supplements, especially calcium, can cure and prevent disease.

Calcium and General Health

In 1994, the National Institutes of Health held a consensus development conference on optimal calcium intake (Optimal Calcium Intake, NIH Consensus Statement Vol. 12, No. 4, June 6- 8, 1994). This conference brought together a group of distinguished experts from several healthcare fields, with the predictable absence of a member from the alternative and complementary medicine field. The conference was notable in defining the answers to several questions.

At the NIH conference, it was *concluded that dietary supplementation with calcium may help prevent osteoporosis.* Osteoporosis was estimated to affect at least 25 million U.S. citizens. Calcium was clearly identified as an essential dietary element that plays a pivotal role in the achievement of a peak bone mass in the first three decades of life. Calcium supplementation modifies the rate of bone loss in later life in conjunction with several other factors. It is clear that optimal calcium intake varies throughout a person's life, with extra needs for calcium occurring during accelerated body growth or pregnancy.

It is very important to realize that a threshold of calcium retention by the body occurs. This calcium retention plays a role in calcium balance. Increases in calcium intake result in retention of calcium by the body, but a level of intake occurs at which increasing intake has no further effect on the incorporation of calcium in the body. The important issue is that calcium supplies need to be abundant in continuity in the diet. The concept of calcium balance is very important in relationship to the maintenance of peak bone mass. When peak bone mass is achieved in men and women around the age of 30 years, the formation of new bone (involving calcium deposition) and the loss of bone (involving calcium removal or re-absorption) become balanced. This balance frequently becomes disturbed in women around the time of the menopause (and in men around andropause), when bone loss tends to occur.

Andropause and Menopause

Bone loss that results in loss of bone density and decrease in peak bone mass occurs synchronously with a decline in body estrogens, which occurs with menopausal onset. The levels of circulating estrogens decrease for 5 to 10 years after the cessation of menstrual periods, and it is believed that this results in bone loss that may not be reversed by increasing calcium intake alone. However, at this stage, the early postmenopausal female is strongly advised to maintain an optimal calcium intake to at least reach the threshold at which maximum calcium incorporation can occur into bone. I believe this intake level is at least 1,500 mg/day for healthy women. *Reader's Digest* reported that the Metabolic Bone Center at St. Lukes Hospital believes that *"a chronic deficiency of calcium is largely responsible for premenstrual syndrome (PMS)"* and that *"a lot of women are avoiding the sun and their vitamin D levels may be very low."*

Several physicians and nutritional scientists are

convinced that the estrogenic components of soy-based diets, which are very high in calcium, are effective in controlling many of the unpleasant symptoms that occur during the menopause. In his book, *The Food Medicine Bible* (1994), Earl Mindell states, *"For example, Japanese women — who eat lots of tofu, bean sprouts and other soya products — rarely complain of menopausal symptoms such as hot flashes, which are quite common among Western women."* He further notes that millions of Western women take pharmaceuticals containing synthetic estrogens to alleviate menopausal symptoms and points out the problem that synthetic estrogens may cause cancer, whereas the isoflavones in soy do not. Similar propositions have been made by Dr. Stephen Holt MD who has also stressed the role of calcium and magnesium intake which selected phytochemicals for menopausal health. These recommendations are highly consistent with the importance of coral calcium as a nutraceutical.

The Digest reported that "in 1997 the large federally financed trial found that a diet containing *1,200 milligrams of calcium significantly lowered blood pressure in adults"*. Then the May 3, 1999 edition of US World News Report wrote in an article entitled *"Calcium's Powerful Mysterious Ways,"* that, *"Researchers are increasingly finding that the humble mineral calcium plays a major role in warding off major illnesses from high blood pressure to colon cancer"* and that *"You name the disease, and calcium is beginning to have a place there"* (David McCarron, a nephrologist at Oregon Health Sciences University). Unfortunately, most doctors have not heard the news that their own journals, major newspapers and magazines are reporting that natural supplements, especially calcium, can cure and prevent cancer.

In recent years, there have been numerous articles on calcium and cancer. In the October 13, 1998 issue of *The New York Times* an article appeared entitled, *"Calcium Takes its Place as a Superstar of Nutrients"* in which it reports that a study published in the Journal of the American Medical Association reported that *"increasing calcium induced normal development of the epithelia cells and might also prevent cancer in such organs as the breast, prostate and pancreas."* It also reported that the American Journal of Clinical Nutrition published "virtually no major organ system escapes calcium's influence" and that a research team from the University of Southern California found "adding calcium to the diet lowered the blood pressure in 110 black teenagers." The January 14, 1999 issue of the *Phoenix Republic* wrote in an article entitled, *"Calcium Reduces Tumors"* that the *New England Journal of Medicine* reported, *"adding calcium to the diet can keep you from getting tumors in your large intestine."* Then the February 1999 issue of *Reader's Digest* wrote in an article entitled *"The 'Superstar' Nutrient"* that the *Journal of the American Medical* published, "when the participants consumption reached *1,500 milligrams of calcium a day, cell growth in the colon improved toward normal* (this means that the cancer was reversed)."

Sources and Amounts of Calcium

Dairy products traditionally have been regarded as the obvious source of dietary calcium, but dairy products as a source of calcium have some disadvantages or limitations. Dairy products contain lactose, and lactose intolerance is particularly common in the elderly, and milk allergies have been documented in up to 20 percent of patients visiting a nutritionally oriented physician. These factors limit the use of dairy products as an efficient source of calcium. Lactose-free products are often unpalatable and expensive. The real negative aspect of milk or dairy product supplementation of the diet is the extra saturated fat and cholesterol load that is provided to an individual. I recommend the use of dairy products, but only to those who like dairy products. Those who do not like milk already are resisting the intake of lactic acid in their already mineral deficient, and therefore acidic bodies, and should only drink milk with some moderation to avoid hypercholesterolemia. However, it should be noted that the British Medical Research Council recently completed a *10-year study* that looked at the health of *5,000 men* aged between 45 and 59. *Only one percent* of those who regularly drank more than one-half liter (about one-half U.S. quart) of milk a day suffered heart attacks in the study period, against *ten percent* of those who drank *no milk at all* (a *tenfold* reduction). Also, drinking more than the one-half of a liter further reduced the incidence of heart attack. Dr. Ann Fehily, one of the team of researchers, states that *"the association between milk drinking and lower heart attack risk was **absolutely clear,** and there was no significance about what type of milk: full, semi-skimmed or full-skimmed."* Thus, the essential ingredient was calcium. Also, a 25-year study ending in 1997 by the Finland National Public Health Institute on 4,697 cancer-free women aged 15 to 90, concluded that there was ***"an overwhelming association between the high consumption of milk and the prevention of breastcancer compared to other factors (WOW!!!)."***

Our literature has recently been full of studies *"suggesting"* that milk consumption is harmful. One such article, found on the internet, *"Calcium in Milk Linked to Prostate Cancer,"* demonstrates the lack of scientific credibility missing in such articles. First, the author did not put his name on the article. Second, the amount of prostate cancer developed on a group of physicians was 4.8% with the "suggested rate of prostate cancer increase" due to milk consumption the study was 30%. This 30% increase, by itself is insignificant because of the small numbers involved in the study. Also, there are numerous factors, which the author of the article was unaware of, that cause an increase in cancer, and unless you evaluate *"all"* of the factors, especially the overriding factors, the study becomes useless. For example, if you are studying the cause of high gas consumption, you could conclude that aerodynamics is the reason. However, if you do not include the overriding factors, i.e.: weight of the vehicles, then your conclusions will be incorrect. The overriding cause of cancer is acidosis, and I am sure that if all of the factors are included, there will be a viable explanation. In addition, the men in the study were physicians who get very little sunshine, which is the overriding factor in calcium absorption (and acidosis). That is why *4.8*% developed prostate cancer. This figure is about 20 times (or *2,000*% more than) the national average. This is a staggering difference that should have been explained, instead of the 30% variation within the figures. If 30% of this staggering 2,000% figure was blamed on milk, what was the 70% of this staggering 2,000% figure blamed on. The anomaly is so high, that it is the overriding factor and requires an explanation before any conclusions can be drawn. I believe that logic dictates that you should be trying to explain a 2,000% anomaly before you discuss a 30% anomaly. The real question should be, "Why did the physicians in this study have a 20-fold increase in prostate cancer?" My conclusion is that physicians get sick due to their diet, lack of milk, lifestyle, and lack of sunshine. In conclusion, those who claim that dairy products do more harm than good can be easily defeated by the facts. God made dairy. God bless dairy.

In his publication, *Homogenized,* the author, Nicholas Sampsidis, tries to prove his contention that the homogenization of milk, which produces a substance called xanthine oxidase (XO), is the main culprit in heart disease. However, the same logic he uses to demonstrate that cholesterol is not guilty (cholesterol threw the last snowball but was the only one to get caught, can also be used to argue that XO is also innocent. When the death rate is factored in with the total milk consumption, a much clearer picture occurs (see table below) which clearly validates Sampsidis' contention that homogenization results in a higher death rate, while invalidating his suggestion that high milk consumption leads to a high death rate. The data clearly shows that high milk consumption reduces the death rate.

Note:
The countries with the highest rate of milk consumption also have the lowest rate of heart disease-induced death (Table 16). France with a low consumption of milk is an exception for lower *"death rate versus milk consumption"* because of the well documented benefits to the heart of its high consumption of wine and because of the higher exposure to sun. At the other end of the scale, the other exception Japan, which apparently has the lowest death rate, has the highest "death rate versus milk consumption" despite its very low homogenization rate due to its extremely low consumption of milk and the fact that its people rarely sunbathe.

144

TABLE 16: Death Rate/Milk Consumption
(Death Rate Per 100,000 and Milk Consumption in Pounds)

Country	Percent Homogenized	Death Rate	Milk Consumption	Death Rate/ Milk Consumption
France	2%	41.9	230	0.18
Sweden	2%	74.7	374	0.20
Switzerland	3%	75.9	370	0.21
Austria	3%	88.6	327	0.27
Netherlands	5%	106.9	337	0.32
U.K.	8%	140.9	350	0.40
Finland	90%	244.7	593	0.41
W. Germany	15%	102.3	213	0.48
Italy	13%	78.9	137	0.57
Canada	13%	187.	4 288	0.65
Australia	50%	204.6	304	0.67
U.S.	95%	211.6	273	0.78
Japan	5%	39.	1 48	0.81

What makes these studies tragic is that they meet all of the prerequisites for scientific authentication that is apparently required by the AMA and yet both studies go unheeded, despite the fact that heeding them could potentially reduce the death rate of heart disease, by *tenfold*, thereby saving millions of lives, as well as providing a means for women to prevent cancer. The fortunate drug companies, and the doctors of America, reap hundreds of billions of dollars per year because of this AMA indifference to using milk nutrition to prevent heart disease and also caustic nutrition to prevent cancer. This indifference, the result of ignorance about nutrition, is also paid for with human suffering as well as hundreds of thousands of lives each year.

Calcium Absorption is Superior from Coral Calcium

The most important issues concerning dietary supplements of minerals and elements relay to their absorbability. Arguments have become prominent among manufacturers of different mineral supplements who claim that one form of mineral or element is better absorbed than another. I believe that the mineral intake of many Western societies is far too low and in the case of calcium and magnesium this intake is falling short of levels that are required for health. It is more than 30 years since a recognition of the importance of the ratio of calcium to magnesium in the promotion of health are particularly cardiac wellness. Reports of the importance of a calcium to magnesium ratio of 2:1 for cardiac health have been repeated in nutritional literature many times in the past decade. This important information prompted scientists at the University of Ryukyus and The University of Okinawato examine carefully the absorption of calcium and other minerals from natural coral calcium.

Experiments at these universities in Japan compared the absorption of calcium from different sources including natural marine based coral calcium, milk derived calcium and cow bone derived calcium (hydroxyapatite). In order to make comparisons, the scientists adjusted the calcium and magnesium ratios in each of these sources of calcium. In the case of marine based coral calcium, no major adjustments were necessary because of the natural 2:1 calcium to magnesium ratio.

To look carefully at calcium absorption, experiments in animals had to be performed. These exhaustive experiments took one month in each group of animals that were fed different types of calcium in their diet. These feeding experiments were carefully controlled and the blood and organs of the animals were examined to measure their calcium and magnesium content. The researchers were focused on the role of calcium and magnesium ratios in heart disease prevention and this made them perform detailed measurements of cholesterol and other fats in the blood.

The results with natural, marine coral were striking. *The amount of calcium found in the animals that were fed with coral calcium was higher than in any other group.* It was notable that the absorption of calcium from coral calcium was approximately 70%, much higher when compared with the other groups of animals who took milk calcium, cow bone calcium or regular calcium supplements. Measurements of blood show that calcium and magnesium levels were similar in each group, regardless of the source of calcium. This observation was not surprising and it reinforces how misleading blood levels of minerals may be as a measure of the overall mineral contents of the body. Clearly, in these experiments natural coral calcium seems to be promoting calcium content of the whole body of the experimental animals.

A clear conclusion from these experiments is that *natural coral calcium seems to be better absorbed* than milk calcium, bone-derived calcium or regular mineral types of calcium. Of major interest in these studies was the observation that the good form of cholesterol (HDL cholesterol) was higher in the animals fed natural coral calcium. This observation is very important because it provides a clue to one important mechanism for the cardiovascular protective effects of coral calcium which occur as a result of the excellent absorption of calcium and presumably other minerals or trace elements from natural coral calcium of marine origin.

Many popular accounts of coral calcium and its health benefits allege that minerals are well absorbed, but these studies provided scientific evidence that coral calcium was an efficient source of mineral. It should be understood that researchers studied marine coral with its naturally occurring ratio of calcium to magnesium of 2:1. It is not known if fossilized coral can produce the same beneficial effects with such promising elements of favorable effect on blood cholesterol.

Arthritis and Osteoporosis Go Hand in Hand

Arthritis and osteoporosis are major public health concerns that often remain recalcitrant to conventional medical interventions. Osteoporosis is a disease of bone that is characterized by a diminution in bone tissue mass per unit volume. This bone thinning results in weakness of the skeleton and a predisposition to bone fractures. In individuals with osteoporosis bone resorption appears to be increased, whereas bone formation may be normal or defective.

The amount of calcium required for the treatment or prevention of osteoporosis appears still to be in dispute (RDA 1.5 g/day), and there have been considerable differences of opinion concerning the format in which dietary calcium supplements should be administered or taken. The relative advantages of one type of calcium supplement versus another often have been reduced to a discussion of the amount of available or absorbable calcium in the product. These arguments may be less important than the other added nutrient advantages of a dietary supplement. For example, nutrient products such as coral calcium provide other essential micronutrients that play a role in bone metabolism, bone calcification, and healthy skeletal structure and function.

Osteoporosis goes *"hand in hand with osteoarthritis"* in many people. Osteoarthritis is primarily a disease affecting hyaline cartilage and adjacent bones. In more advanced cases of osteoarthritis the tissue in and around the joints becomes hypertrophic. Damaged by a line cartilage break, fissures and develops an irregular surface in the osteoarthritic joint, where friction often causes crepitus (creaking) of joints. Osteoarthritis seems to occur invariably with advancing age. It is the most common form of arthritis and it is universal in males and females after the age of 65 years, even though it may be asymptomatic.

Both osteoporosis and osteoarthritis have poorly defined etiologies (Tables 1, 2 and 3). Recent research has implicated nutritional factors as important in the maintenance of bone and joint health. Despite the increasing recognition that osteoarthritis and osteoporosis may have nutritional abnormalities at the root of their causation, dietary manipulations have often played a secondary role in the management of these diseases. Recently, nutritional interventions have been increasingly proposed as potentially effective options for arthritis and thin bones (osteoporosis).

Table 17

Some of the Factors in the Etiology of Osteoarthritis. The Most Common Factors Contributing to Osteoarthritis in Western Society are Advancing Age, Poor Nutrition, Trauma and Obesity. Minerals and Elements Play a Major Role in Maintaining the Health of Bones and Cartilage

Causative Factor	Comment— Circumstance
Genetics heredofamilial tendencies.	Heberden's nodes Postural defects, Idiopathic generalized osteoarthritis.
Crystalline deposition in joints	Uric acid Calcium pyrophosphate and hydroxyapatite.
Advanced age	Defects in collagen structure in cartilage, spontaneous cartilage fractures, diminished aggregation of proteoglycans, lack of resilience of supporting tissues, abnormal anatomical circumstances.
Repetitive stress	Excessive sports activity, coexistent neuropathy, muscular dystrophy.
Poor nutrition	Deficiency of antioxidants, key vitamins and minerals that are important for metabolic function in chondrocytes and matrix formation of cartilage.

Metabolic diseases	Acromegaly, copper storage disease, ochronosis.
Eccentric mechanical stress	Joint instability, hypermobility, previous trauma to cartilage, postural defects abnormal joint development, obesity.
Previous joint infection	Syphilis, Gonoccal arthritis Pyogenic arthritis.

Types of Osteoporosis and Osteoarthritis

Osteoporosis is a common phenomenon in the postmenopausal and post- andropausal adult. This type of osteoporosis has been termed Type 1 and it is up to ten times more common in females than in males. Type 1 osteoporosis tends to effect cancellous bones such as the vertebral column and it has been repeatedly linked to hormonal changes that occur in the postmenopausal female, most notably estrogen deficiency. The importance of the life-long deficiency of calcium in causing this disorder may have been somewhat underestimated. In contrast, Type II osteoporosis (senile osteoporosis) is more related to nutritional factors such as deficiency of vitamin D or resistance to the bone related effects of this vitamin. Dietary calcium deficiency is of significant importance in the causation of senile osteoporosis and this makes the contents of coral calcium particularly useful as a dietary supplement to support bone and joint health.

Table 18
Risk Factors Described for Primary Osteoporosis

- Female sex
- Premature menopause
- Advanced age
- Race (more common in whites)
- Lifelong calcium deficiency
- Lack of exercise
- Genetic predisposition
- Ectomorphic build
- Nulliparity
- Low phytonutrient intake
- Trace metal deficiency

In common with Type 1 osteoporosis, Type II osteoporosis is generally more common in females but the apparent increased prevalence of this disorder may be related to the fact that women live longer than men. A number of risk factors for Type 1 and Type II osteoporosis have been identified. These are summarized in Table 2. Osteoporosis can be secondary to a variety of readily identifiable causes (Table 3) but secondary osteoporosis accounts for less than one in twenty of all cases of all forms of osteoarthritis. Type 1 and Type II osteoporosis may occur together and in some circumstances they may be exacerbated by some of the causes of secondary osteoporosis that are listed in Table 3. Hence, the causation of osteoporosis is multi-factorial (many different mechanisms), thereby dictating the need for multiple treatment interventions. The intervention that is common to help all types of osteoporosis is calcium and minerals in the diet.

Table 19

Causes of Secondary Osteoporosis

Drug Induced:

Alcohol, tobacco, barbiturates, phenytoin, heparin and cortico steroids.

Endocrine Disorders:

Diabetes mellitus, excess glucocorticoids, hyperparathyroidism, hyperthyroidism, hypogonadism, hyperprolactinemia.

Miscellaneous Factors:

Lack of exercise (especially immobilization), kidney disease, arthritis (interfering with locomotor ability), cancer, liver disease, intestinal disease (causing malabsorption) and chronicpulmonary disorders.

Connie W. Bales Ph.D. and her colleagues from Duke University Medical Center indicate that the lifetime risk of a woman to develop a hip fracture is much greater in the presence of osteoporosis. This risk is equal to a woman's combined risk of developing ovarian, uterine and breast cancer. This devastating projection is even worse when one considers the fact that elderly people often die shortly after the occurrence of a fractured hip or they remain bed-bound in their terminal years of life. Thus, osteoporosis which is caused by mineral deficiency to a major degree is a lethal disease that often destroys the quality of life of the elderly.

The link between nutrition and osteoarthritis is less

clear than it is in the case of osteoporosis (Table 19 and 20). However, contemporary thinking has been directed to the consideration that osteoarthritis be related, in part, to *"malnourished"* cartilage. Osteoarthritis has been classified as primary or secondary to a variety of causes. Several etiologic factors may act in a synergistic manner in the causation of joint disease (Table 20).

The common causes of secondary osteoarthritis are highlighted in Table 19. It is believed that the most common form of osteoarthritis may be related in part to the "wear and tear" of joints. The recognition that osteoarthritis is a disease of cartilage has precipitated research into the many mechanisms that could alter the microenvironment of cartilage and factors that nourish and protect the tissue from damage. Minerals and elements are among the most important nourishing factors in the diet that can determine skeletal health.

Table 20
Factors That May Cause Secondary Osteoarthritis

- Trauma to joints and adjacent fracture of bones.
- Metabolic and endocrine disease.
- Neuropathic disease.
- Congenital disorders of joints.
- Secondary to other types of arthritis e.g. rheumatoid disease.
- Overuse of joints.
- Infections of joints.

Achieving Optimal Bone Density

Age affects bone mass and joint mobility. Peak bone mass is reached in males and females between the age of 20 and 30 years. It is known that the level of bone density at the time of peak bone mass is an important factor for determining bone health throughout the later years of life. Individuals in Western society lose up to 0.5 % of bone mass on an annual basis and this reduction in bone density accelerates after menopause. The reductions in bone mass that occur with age can be reduced by optimal nutrition, especially adequate mineral and trace element intake.

Good nutrition undoubtedly plays a major role in determining the achievement of optimal bone density but weight-bearing exercise is a proven way of increasing bone density, even without any form of therapy, nutritional or otherwise. The author believes that many accounts of the prevention or treatment of osteoporosis and osteoarthritis fail to recognize the importance of a regular program of exercise that involves repeated muscular activity against gravity. Weight-bearing exercise is germane to the success of the treatment or prevention of both osteoarthritis and osteoporosis. Studies of populations with longevity show a tendency for regular exercise in the lifetime of these elite elderly.

More Focus on Calcium and Osteoporosis

It is important to further review matters concerning calcium and bone health. Calcium is the principle cationic element found in bone mineral and without adequate dietary intake of calcium adequate bone mass cannot be achieved. It is known that calcium deficiency in early life is associated with an increased risk of fracture, even in adolescence, and it has a strong association with the occurrence of osteoporosis in the mature adult. Calcium requirements vary throughout life and dietary intake of calcium is highly related to the development of optimal bone mass during life.

Life-long calcium deficiency is a very important, widely accepted cause of osteoporosis, but calcium does not work effectively in the absence of the minerals and elements. Several studies have reported favorable reductions in bone loss in postmenopausal women who have received calcium, vitamin D, or estrogen replacement therapy alone or in combination. Other studies, using multiple nutrient therapy with calcium and minerals as a focus of treatment, have produced similar beneficial results in the treatment of osteoporosis. Important studies using calcium supplementation of the diet have indicated a reduction in the prevalence of osteoporotic vertebral crush fractures in postmenopausal women. Estrogen supplements are given to postmenopausal women to reduce menopausal symptoms and, arguably, to promote cardiovascular health and reduce osteoporosis. However, estrogen and other synthetic hormonal supplements have unfortunate adverse effects and risks, such as the promotion of uterine and breast cancer and peripheral venous thrombosis.

The beneficial effects of calcium supplementation on bone loss in premenopausal and postmenopausal *"middle-aged women"* is well recognized. A study by

Dawson-Hughes M.D. and his colleagues (1987) showed that women had a loss of bone density when they had a daily calcium consumption of less than 400mg/day. Loss of bone density was much less in those women who had a calcium intake of approximately 750mg/day. Although some other studies have failed to show a major beneficial effect of calcium supplementation in preventing or reversing osteoporosis, an overwhelming body of opinion is in favor of calcium supplementation as a preventive measure for osteoporosis. Table 21 shows the NIH recommendations for optimal calcium intake, but I believe that these recommendations are underestimates. Given the well-described role of calcium in bone health, one may wonder why the relationship between calcium intake and osteoporosis is not crystal clear in all studies. The reason is simple and it relates to the absolute requirement of many other minerals and trace elements. The varied mineral and trace element content of coral calcium explains why bone health is common in Okinawa and other longevous populations that have abundant nutrient elements in their environment (e.g. Hunzas).

Table 21
Optimal Calcium Requirements During an Individual's Lifetime

This data is taken from NIH Consensus Statement, Vol.12, No.4, June 6-8, 1994.

Stage of Life	Optimal Daily Intake (in mg of calcium)
Women	
25-50 years	1,000
Pregnant and nursing	1,200-1,500
Over 50 years postmenopausal	
On estrogens	1,000

Not on estrogens	1,500
Over 65 years	1,500

Men

25-65 years	1,000
Over 65 years	1,500

Adolescents/Young Adults

11-24 years	1,200-1,500

Children

Up to 10 years	800-1,200

Infants

Up to 1 year	400-600

Note: These estimates, which have undergone dramatic increases over the years, have been raised upwards in some circumstances and I believe that there is evidence to even further increase recommended intakes of calcium, as most long-living cultures consume over 100 times these amounts recommended.

The treatment of established osteoporosis is even more disappointing in outcome than the treatment of oster-arthritis using conventional medical therapy. Not enough attention has been paid to the prevention of osteoporosis, despite the realization that its occurrence is universal in the elderly. Acute or chronic pain as a result of osteoporotic fractures is often treated by NSAID (non-steroidal anti-inflammatory drugs) and adjunctive physical therapy or the application of cumbersome, orthopedic garments. These interventions are necessitated by repeated bone fractures or the common coexistence of osteoarthritis with osteoporosis. Calcium supplementation for men or women with osteoporosis with or without vitamin D supplements is commonly used to treat osteoporosis but it has questionable efficacy and the attendant risk of producing hypercalcemia, especially since these patients rarely get the exposure to sunshine that is necessary to produce the calcium regulators, calcitonin and inisotol triphosphate. It should be noted that S. Kawamura, in his book *Warning! Calcium Deficiency* based on 20,000 case histories over 30 years, discovered that some of the 40 over-the-counter calcium products, especially liquid ionized calcium, resulted in hypercalcemia. He also discovered that when the patients ingested coral calcium or other marine calcium products, none developed hypercalcemia.

In the book *Molecular and Cellular Regulation of Calcium and Phosphate Metabolism,* 1990 Alan R. Liss Inc., Dr. Meunier writes an article entitled *Treatment of Vertebral Osteoporosis,* in which he concludes *"When calcium and vitamin D is given in daily doses along with moderate amounts of sodium fluoride to patients with osteoporosis, there is a substantial increase in bone mass and a **significant reduction** in the incidence of further vertebral fractures."*

In the book *The Calcium Factor,* Barefoot states, *"the calcium deposits in the tissues and joints of older people is also a sign of the calcium regulatory system adjusting to a severe calcium deficiency. The bony deposits reduce movement and cause pain and thereby limit activity in order to bolster the sagging skeletal structural strength resulting from the osteoporosis or decalcification of the bones.*

*These **calcium deposits**, which are a **direct result of calcium deficiency**, ironically enhance the fear of increasing calcium consumption, which would alleviate and correct the problem. Thus, some of the many diseases that are related to the last resort removal of calcium from the bones are osteoporosis, arthritis, rheumatism, sclerosis, and periodontal disease."*

Barefoot also notes that osteoporosis is a major problem in space flights. He states, *"It is known that **space flight osteoporosis**, decalcification of up to 8 percent of the bones which occurs after only a few weeks in orbit, is probably **due to the unnatural electrical currents induced in the body**. The rapid motion through the Earth's magnetic field produced these, (the human body, a poor conductor cutting though 37,000 magnetic lines per second thereby generating electrical current in the body) with polarity reversal every half-hour resulting in induced biochemical cellular reactions. It was also known that cell division cycle time, which involves the duplication of all the cells' DNA and the chromosomes that are then distributed equally between two cells, **takes exactly one day**. This implies that **tissue repair**, that depends on regulated cell division, **is synchronized with the Earth's magnetic field**. In the 1960s scientists overcame space osteoporosis by strapping on electromagnetic coils that approximated the bones' normal gravity stress signals, and stimulated cell growth by using pulsed electromagnetic fields at the Schumann rate of resonance that induced currents within the body from outside the body. In 1979, pulsed electromagnetic fields had been demonstrated as so effective in stimulated bone healing of the elderly, that the authorities yielded to pressure and gave their rare approval to have pulsed electromagnetic units installed in every major hospital in America."*

With regard to osteoporosis, Barefoot further states that *"Up to **one-third of all elderly men and women** fracture a hip will accidentally fracture a hip. **Over one-half** of the elderly who end up in a nursing home, and up to one-fifth can die as a result of the accident. The elderly are also very susceptible to fractures of the vertebrae (back bones) and wrists. **Osteoporosis**, which represents adaptive decalcification of the bones, is the culprit. The ignorant use of painkillers will only permit the culprit to survive, worsening the disease until fractures occur. This culprit, like the ones responsible for a host of other diseases, could be shot down with the silver bullet, biological calcium, and **coral calcium** is the best calcium nutrient known to man."*

Preventing Osteoporosis

Scientific literature often focuses on the prevention and therapy of osteoporosis, but overall the results of treatment of established osteoporosis are disappointing. Contemporary literature draws attention to alternative medical and primary nutrient approach to osteoporosis therapy. The possibility that sugar, caffeine, salt and alcohol and other potentially harmful dietary constituents promote osteoporosis is very plausible and backed by scientific evidence. In addition to the relatively poor nutrient value of processed foods, poor soil quality and pollution of farmland are factors that determine the inadequate nutrient value of crops. This latter problem is abolished in many longevous communities, such as Okinawa, where the soil and water is enriched with minerals from coral calcium.

A Symphony of Nutrients

A whole host of other dietary factors and micronutrients may play a variable part in promoting skeletal health, including vitamins K, B6, C and D, manganese, magnesium, folic acid, strontium, boron, zinc, copper and silicon. Calcium, phosphorus and vitamin D appear to play the most important role in maintaining a healthy skeletal function, compared with all of these other dietary factors. These nutrients work as a symphony to build bones and joints.

Table 22
Nutrients Required in a Balanced Diet for Bone, and Perhaps Joint Health. Proposed by Stephen Holt, M.D.

Nutrient	Comment
Calcium	Unequivocal evidence for benefit.
Fluoride	Trace amounts are beneficial, over inclusion damages bones.
Silica	Enhances bone mineralization and function of bone collagen.
Zinc	Facilitates calcium absorption and is necessary for enzyme systems in matrix building, antioxidant properties.
Manganese	Essential role in cartilage and collagen formation in the skeleton.

Boron	Facilitates calcium and magnesium utilization and function.
Magnesium	Facilitates calcium, vitamin D and hormonal effects on bones.
Phosphorus	Combines with calcium in salts in bones and is vital for many cellular functions.
Copper	Facilitates collagen and matrix synthesis.
Soy Isoflavones	Striking recent evidence for benefit in osteoporosis.
Vitamins A,B3,B6, C,D,B 12,K,Folate	Vitamin D is the most important regulator of calcium and phosphorus metabolism. B3 and B6 are enzymatic cofactors in collagen metabolism. Vitamin A is vital in osteoblast function and it regulates calcium metabolism. Vitamin C is vital for healthy collagen synthesis. Vitamin K is necessary for osteocalcin synthesis, the matrix upon which calcium is deposited in bone. B12 promotes chondrocytic and osteoblastic metabolism. Folate is antihomocysteine, thereby being antiosteoporotic and antiatherosclerotic.
Essential Fatty Acids	Essential for calcium metabolism and cell membrane function. The ratio of Omega 3 to Omega 6 fatty acids is distorted in Western diets. Many diets are Omega 3 deficient.

Our U.S. Food Pyramid

The classic guidelines of the Food Guide Pyramid are not adequate for individuals who are at risk of osteoporosis. Dr. Connie W. Bales and her colleagues from Duke University in North Carolina have recommended that these existing dietary guidelines of 2 or 3 daily servings of dairy products be replaced by 4 or 5 daily servings of low-fat, dairy products to increase the daily intake of calcium, in order to prevent osteoporosis. The author proposes that there are more efficient dietary maneuvers that will prevent osteoporosis without resorting to unhealthy enhanced intake of dairy products. Such maneuvers include the use of coral calcium as a supplement and the avoidance of the *"calcium-wasting"* effects of excessive animal protein.

Switching to Vegetable-Based Diets

There seem to be several compelling reasons to switch from animal protein diets to fruit and vegetable diets that are rich in vitamins, minerals and other nutrients in order to achieve optimal bone and joint health. Examples of these benefits are most apparent particularly when one examines the benefits of certain phytonutrient (phyto means plant) fractions of certain legumes, such as soybeans. It is recognized that soy protein inclusion in diets may promote calcium retention in the body. In contrast, animal protein may tend to increase calcium excretion in the urine, lower urinary citrate excretion and increase uric acid excretion. As well as a negative impact on bone health, these circumstances may lead to a tendency to form urinary calculi (stones).

P. Kontessis M.D. and his colleagues studied the renal, metabolic, and hormonal responses to animal and vegetable protein diets and observed enhancement of renal the function with the use of a vegetable protein diet. This clinical investigation showed the greater efficiency with which the human kidney can handle vegetable protein compared with the efficiency of handling animal protein. It was found that glomerular filtration rate was about one-fifth higher after the dietary inclusion of animal protein than after soy protein.

Fruit and vegetable diets can deliver a vast array of health-giving phytonutrients that have versatile health giving benefits, including anticancer effects and antioxidant effects. Of particular importance in some vegetarian diets is the presence of soy isoflavones (genistein, daidzein and glycitein) from soybeans. These phytonutrients have been shown to prevent and treat osteoporosis in controlled studies in animals and humans.

Vitamins and Trace Elements

Several minerals and vitamins play a major role in metabolic processes that produce and the matrix of bone and cartilage. Conventional medicine has not focused much attention on the importance of micronutrients in the synthesis of supporting components of bone or cartilage, despite the clear recognition that diets deficient in several micronutrients cause multiple bone lesions in animals. Benefit is apparent in bone integrity when trace minerals such as manganese and zinc are added to calcium supplementation of the diet. These findings have major implications for the use of coral calcium and the formulation of other dietary supplements. Nutraceuticals for bone and joint health are effective when they contain selected trace minerals.

Vitamins K and C play pivotal roles in the metabolism of bone and cartilage. Vitamin K deficiency is not uncommon in the elderly as a consequence of poor dietary intake or reduced colonic synthesis of this vitamin by normal bacteria the colon. Vitamin K is obligatory in the enzymatic formation of bone matrix proteins and Vitamin C enhances the cross-linking of collagen, which can only occur with the supply of essential mineral and element nutrients. It is clear that supplementation of these two vitamins alone may be beneficial in many circumstances in the elderly, but this option may be forgotten frequently. The obvious value of vitamin D and C is why they are added to coral calcium formulas that I recommend as dietary supplements.

Vitamin D has unequivocal importance in bone health and levels of 25 hydroxy-vitamin D (25,O,H,D) fall with age. Dairy milk that is sold in the US is fortified with vitamin D to give approximately 100 IUs per serving, but soymilk fortified with vitamin D is also available. The author believes that calcium and vitamin D-fortified soymilk, are ideal for the promotion of bone health because of their valuable content of soy isoflavones.

Clarifying Recommendations for Diet

Both dietary excesses and dietary inadequacies play a role in bone health and general well-being. The concept of the balanced diet for bones and joints is worth summarizing by considering many of the most important nutrients for skeletal health (Table 22). The switch towards a vegetarian diet does not necessarily need to be complete to promote bone health. A well-balanced omnivorous diet can be healthy, provided that animal protein and fat intake is limited.

The average Western diet is characteristically too high in cholesterol, saturated fat and animal protein. Dairy products have been overemphasized as an important dietary component for healthy bones and teeth. Dairy products may precipitate milk protein allergy and they often deliver a high caloric and high, saturated fat load. Alternative sources of calcium in the diet from fish and green vegetables together with coral calcium provide an ideal way of supplementing calcium and valuable minerals in the diet.

A balanced diet for bone health should limit caffeine, alcohol, simple sugar, saturated fat, excessive animal protein, and excessive phosphorus. Each of these elements of Western diets have been shown to exert one or more deleterious effects on the bone and joint health. The Western diet often contains too many calories, derived especially from fat (as much as 150-180 gm of fat per day in Europe and the USA). Calorie restriction is of pivotal importance in weight reduction and low energy density foods are to be preferred in many cases.

The switch to vegetables in the diet often achieves calorie restriction in a gradual and comfortable manner. Vegetables can promote satiety because of their relatively low calorie bulk and fiber content. Dietary fiber promotes health in general but care is advised with excessive intake of coarse fiber, such as bran, which can limit calcium absorption. The effective treatment of obesity alone is often very successful in the management of osteoarthritis in weight-bearing joints and preventing fractures in osteoporotic bones.

Chapter Summary

Nobody can promise cure of established bone and joint disease by diet alone but nutritional therapies provide the greatest hope and remain an area of neglect in many conventional and some alternative therapies for arthritis and osteoporosis. Recent research has pointed the way to an optimal diet for the prevention and treatment of bone and joint disorders, where adequate mineral and trace element intake plays a special role.

Despite advances in knowledge about the importance of nutrition for skeletal health, the general practice of medicine, conventional, integrated or alternative, remains often unable, or unwilling of applying innovative nutritional approaches to the management of osteoporosis. Enactment of more universal nutritional approaches to osteoporosis and osteoarthritis will pave the way to the eradication of these diseases. Mineral supplements make perfect sense as an important supplement for healthy bones given their inadequate intake in the average Western diet, and coral calcium figures as an important natural dietary supplement.

CHAPTER 9

<u>Body Acidity, Alkalinity,</u>
<u>Minerals and Health</u>

The Concept and Biological Importance of Body pH

Modern medicine has focused a great deal of effort on understanding the importance of acidity and alkalinity as factors that control body chemistry. Medical textbooks contain complex information on how to correct gross disturbances of acid-base (alkali) balance, but few discuss the role of subtle controls of acidity on health and well-being. Considerable evidence exists that a standard Western diet often leads to a chronic state of low-level acidosis (acidity of the body). For example, a healthy patient will have a saliva pH of 7.5, while a cancer patient will have a saliva pH of 4.5, or *1,000 times as much acid*. This continuing body acidity contributes to poor health. It is important to understand how this body acidity is created, and that except for the stomach acid and urine, all body fluids are kept acidic by minerals, especially calcium. Several sources of an acidic load to the body include diet (lack of minerals), stress resulting in excessive cortisol and adrenaline secretion in the body and continuing insults to the immune system. It should be noted that since the consumption of calcium leads to the termination of acidosis, then the consumption of coral, providing 50 times as much 50 times as fast, can be extremely effective.

Acidity and alkalinity are measured by a logarithm scale, referred to as pH. The concept of pH confuses many people. This log scale of measurement of acidity and alkalinity means that a small change in pH results from a large change (tenfold) in hydrogen or hydroxyl ion concentrations. The dictionary defines an acid as one of a group of substances that neutralize or are neutralized by alkalies. This definition may help to class a group of substances, as either acids or alkalies, but for the average person, it does not explain what either substance truly is. The chemical dictionary defines acid as one of a large class of chemicals that has the property of ionizing or splitting of the water molecule, H-O-H, to produce positive hydronium ions, more commonly referred to as hydrogen ions, (H)+. In contrast, an alkali is a chemical that splits water producing the negative hydroxyl ion, (OH)-. Thus, acids are substances that ionize to give a solvent an excess of the positive hydrogen ion, and alkalies are substances that ionize to give a solvent the negative hydroxyl ion. The concentration of these ions, acidity and alkalinity, are described as numbers, pH values, that are logarithmic (to the base ten) reflections. When the number of alkaline (OH)- ions present in a fluid equals that of the acidic (H)+ ions, the fluid is in the neutral state and its pH is 7.0. Increases in acidic (H)+ ions produce changes from 7 to 14. It is important to remember that the intervals on the pH scale are exponential. Therefore the pH scale represents vastly wider differences in concentration than the figures themselves seem to indicate. A pH change of one unit reflects a ten-fold change in the hydrogen ion or the hydroxyl ion concentration.

More About Acids, Alkalies and Minerals

It is therefore apparent that ionization occurs in both acidic and alkaline solutions. The digestive system is made more efficient by the fact that most foods are acidic, thereby generating their own acids and thus requiring less acid from the body for total digestion. Some examples of the pH and acidity or alkalinity of certain foods are given in Table 23.

Table 23: Food and pH

FOOD	pH
Lemon	2.1
Vinegar	2.7
Apples	3.1
Grapefruit	3.1
Rhubarb	3.1
Strawberries	3.2
Raspberries	3.4
Tomatoes	4.2
Bananas	4.6
Carrots	5.1
Beans	5.5
Bread	5.5
Asparagus	5.6
Potatoes	5.8
Butter	6.3
Corn	6.3
Shrimp	6.9
Water	7.0
Egg Whites	7.8

During digestion, hydrochloric acid is produced in the stomach and the gastric contents are very acidic, ranging from pH 1 to pH 3. This acid, hydrochloric acid is produced from the consumption of salt, sodium chloride. Recent studies have shown that doubling the salt intake reduces the production of the hormone, renin, which results in a dramatic reduction in heart disease as well as prolonging life. Since almost all minerals containing chlorides are soluble, they remain ionized. The hydrochloric acid secreted by the stomach is a highly effective way of ionizing elements in the food. However, food usually contains products that produce ions other than chlorides, such as the phosphates from meat and soft drinks, the citrates from fruits, and the lactates from milk, to name but a few.

When some of these chemical radicals are present in large numbers in food they present a problem, because they can bond together with other elements to create insoluble compounds that can precipitate. Therefore, many elements are not readily ionizable at the strength of the acid that is in the stomach. An example of this is the precipitation of calcium phosphate, a mineral called "apatite," when the negative phosphate ion comes in contact with the positive calcium ion. The resulting apatite is not absorbed into the body. If however, other anions, such as lactates from milk or malates from apples, are present in sufficient quantities, the calcium in the diet may form significant amounts of calcium lactate and calcium malate, which are both soluble, and they remain ionized, even when they become alkalized in the duodenum. It has to be realized that simple chemical discussions do not take account of the complexities of the digestive process. For example, some calcium is absorbed directly in an ionized form, but much calcium requires the action of vitamin D for optimum absorption from the intestines. The microclimate of the gastrointestinal tract plays a major role in food assimilation and general health of the body.

Eating food, which contains substances that the body craves, is not a good way to maintain health. The average Western taste preference is for sweet food containing excessive amounts of fat. This dietary preference is undoubtedly contributing to poor health and especially to the recent epidemic of diabetes mellitus.

Unfortunately, other pertinent parameters exist that will create an unhealthy state of the body even though apparently nutritious foods are consumed. I believe that the body will crave food of different types to obtain specific nutrients that are required for health. Examples of this type of *"unconscious"* eating behavior has been well documented in animals. For example, the first part of the prey that the tiger or the polar bear eats is the intestines that are full of vegetation. Whilst one may crave fruits and vegetables to get the trace metals that the body requires, deficiency may remain because the particular soil, that was chosen to grow these seemingly nutritious foods, may have been devoid of these required trace metals. It should be understood that when the body consumes, digests and absorbs most of the nutrients it requires, but remains deficient in only one element, the body will remain in an unhealthy state because the cells of the body may not be able to fully utilize nutrients in an efficient manner.

The Real Implications of Body pH for Health

Conventional medicine teaches that gross changes of body pH are highly threatening to health and on occasion they can result in death. Nobody has any difference of opinion, but conventional medicine will not accept wholeheartedly the concept that chronic body acidity is the cause of much disease, even though the acidity means that oxygen will be driven from the body. I have been impressed by one recent article on acid-alkaline balance in the body, that was published in the *International Journal of Integrative Medicine* (2, 6, 2,000) by Drs. S. Brown and R. Jaffe. These authors focus their attention on body pH and its effects on bone health. However, body pH has wide ranging influences on body chemistry and, in term, body structure and function.

In this recent article by Brown and Jaffe, a quotation from the Nobel Prize-winning scientist Dr. A. Szent-Gyrogy was used as a basis to discuss the implications of pH balance in the body. Szent-Gyrogy states, *"the body is alkaline by design but acidic by function."* This profound statement supports my hypotheses on the importance of mineral and element intake in the diet that will favor minor, healthy degrees of body alkalinity.

Brown and Jaffe make a very important observation by stating that *"The human body has also been described as largely dilute seawater encapsulated in a membrane skin."* It is known that the body functions in a tight range of pH and this pH is slightly alkaline. Without detailed discussion, it is clear that adequate nutrient mineral intake is an absolute prerequisite of healthy body function, if only for a simple chemical reason that minerals and selected elements are important controllers of body pH. Thus, all the jazz about coral calcium makes perfect sense in a scientific perspective and we now must recognize how it makes sense to identify abundant mineral and element intake in healthy and longevous populations as an important elixir of life.

Think About Our Lousy Diet and Body pH

The Standard American Diet (SAD) often provides or produces a large amount of acid for the body to deal with (up to 200 mEq per day). Elegant studies on the influence of certain foods on body pH tell a story that must make scientists, physicians, nutritionists and any health conscious person stop and think about the necessity for pH balancing minerals in the diet. In simple terms, body acidity and calcium deficiency are handled by the body's clever ways of surviving. Acid foods with body acidosis and low calcium intake results in immediate release of calcium from its stores in the body. It is now quite simple to understand why many people in Western society have thin bones and rotten teeth.

There are certain trends in our *"fast food nation"* and our *"big gulp society"* that propagate body acidity. These include red meat and carbonated soda (cola) consumption. For example, a diet that contains 120 g of protein per day produces an excretion of acid by the body of about 150 mEq. This is nearly a couple of hamburgers and a popular soft drink. We all know that popular soda drinks are refreshing, but few people think about their highly acidic nature. It has been calculated that fizzy cola or orange crush or lemon crush etc. has a pH on the major acidic side (range pH 2.8-3.1). I believe that we are going to experience continuing acceleration of common chronic diseases e.g. heart disease, cancer and osteoporosis if we do not pay more attention to correcting our tendency to maintain body acidity. The ability of the body to buffer acid is limited by the consumption of nutrients such as calcium and this ability is constantly tested or impaired by common diseases that are determined by adverse diet and lifestyle. Adequate calcium allows the body to produce the buffer calcium mono ortho phosphate (R. Barefoot, *The Calcium Factor*), which with sodium bicarbonate, maintain the body fluids at a pH of 7.4. Without this mechanism, the blood would become acidic and we would die immediately.

Most scientists are not impressed with altering diets to favor acidic versus alkaline foods but what is not discussed is the importance of certain foods in generating acidity in the body. Modern nutritionists are looking for ways to maintain minor degrees of alkalinity and a convenient, rapid and effective way to achieve this is to take coral calcium, whilst increasing vegetable and fruit intake, reducing animal protein intake and avoiding excessive stress. What I have described, is the lifestyle of Okinawans, with the smiling faces of their elite elderly.

Chapter Summary

Talking about pH and chemistry can be a turn off. However, it is recognized that Western living produces a sustained, low level of body acidity. This status causes much disease and poor health. For example, a person in Okinawa has forty times, or so, less chance of osteoporotic fracture than the average person in Western society. I am convinced that one factor accounting for this and other health advantages of Okinawan people is related to coral calcium in their environment. Abundant mineral and element supply may help correct this problem and with other lifestyle measures some chronic disease may be vanquished.

CHAPTER 10

Coral Calcium Facts and Experiences

The Influence of Coral Calcium on Health

Because of the highly varied and essential mineral content of coral calcium, few people are surprised by its potent and versatile health benefits when it is given as a dietary supplement. The importance of the calcium factor for health and longevity was extensively reviewed in chapter 8. Suffice it to say, as the "King of the Bioelements," calcium provides benefit for almost all normal tissue functions in the body, but it needs other minerals and companion trace elements to function in an optimal manner.

Among the many nutrients required by the body for health, minerals possess a chemical power to rejuvenate the chemistry of life. In summary, minerals play a well-defined role in function of the nervous system, contraction of muscles, especially the heart, and they can help overcome fatigue. In addition, minerals play a major role in skin health and hair growth. Without essential minerals many vital body functions are impaired.

Orthomolecular Medicine

Abram Hoffer M.D., Ph.D is the founder of a discipline called orthomolecular medicine. In simple terms this is the supply of the correct compounds (molecules) in correct amounts and forms (ortho). Of particular significance is the work of Dr. Hoffer in substituting drugs with nutritional therapies to treat a variety of diseases including schizophrenia and cardiovascular disease. In his book entitled *Smart Nutrients*, Dr. Hoffer explains how mineral imbalance causes ill health and alters an individual's disposition.

According to Dr. Hoffer, a deficiency minerals leads to fatigue, forgetfulness, lackluster skin and hair, a short temper, nervous tension, defeatism, depression vengefulness and even suicidal tendencies. Dr. Hoffer states, *"In fact, if anyone has a shortage of just one mineral, he can expect that his system will begin to weaken and lose its efficiency, with disease eventually setting in."* (Quoted from *Smart Nutrients*, Hoffer A. and Walker M., Avery Publishing Group, New Canaan, CT, 1994).

The Balance of Minerals in the Body

The biochemistry of how minerals maintain balance is highly complex. All body fluids contain mineral salts that work with cells to maintain electrolyte (chemical balance). We have learned in Chapter 4 that minerals generate minute amounts of electricity. Several authors have likened all cells of the body to small batteries with electrical changes that are governed by mineral (element) movements and contents.

Taking Minerals in the Diet

I reiterate that population studies support the hypothesis that taking minerals in adequate and well regulated quantities will contribute to health and long life.

However, a degree of balance of mineral availability in the body is required. On the one hand there are major classes of dietary minerals (e.g. calcium and magnesium) required in relatively large amounts, whereas on the other there are trace minerals, which are required only in small quantities. Many trace minerals are required for optimum health.

Much literature has appeared on the role of adequate calcium, magnesium and zinc intake on health promotion and the arrest o body aging. Practitioners of conventional and alternative medicine have stressed the advantages of deriving adequate mineral intake in the diet from a generous intake of fruit, vegetables and nuts. I do not deny that this is an ideal approach, but much modern produce may be lacking somewhat in minerals and adults "on the go" or the elderly cannot be meticulous about their dietary habits. Current estimates are that three quarters of the population may have an inadequate intake of calcium, magnesium, vitamin C and trace minerals. For these reasons, coral calcium represents a practical and balanced approach to mineral supplementation of the Western diet.

The clear advantage of coral calcium is the presence of chelated mineral atoms that are surrounded by larger molecules. In this chelated form the charges (electric fields) of the minerals are changed so that they are better absorbed by the body and readily utilized in the vital chemistry of life. Also, the contained marine nutrients are particularly suited to enhance the digestion/absorption in a mineral rich and salty intestine.

Picking Foods with Good Mineral Content

I advise individuals to be knowledgeable about the

mineral content of various foods. Unfortunately, many trace metals are most abundant in more esoteric forms of food that are not easily placed on the average family's dinner menu. Table 25 reviews good sources of minerals and trace minerals that are beneficial for health.

Table 24
Some Common Sources of Major and Trace Minerals. Note that Some of the Most Abundant Sources of Minerals in Foods Came from Uncommon Foods in the Average Diet. Without Meticulous Dietary Planning Isolated Mineral Deficiencies are Common. This is Why Supplements of Minerals and Trace Elements Such as Coral Calcium Make Sense

Mineral/Element	Food In Which Mineral is Abundant
Calcium	Kelp, dairy products, carob flour, collard greens, turnip greens, etc.
Magnesium	Kelp, wheat cereals, nuts (especially almonds), etc.
Phosphorus	Wheat, nuts and seeds, some cheeses.
Sodium	Ubiquitous, biggest source may be table salt added to food.
Potassium	Seeds, wheat, nuts, parsley, beans, etc.
Iron	Kelp, brewer's yeast, wheat, animal liver, parsley, clams, red meat, etc.
Copper	Oysters, nuts, lecithin from soy, animal liver, cod liver oils, etc.

Manganese	Nuts (pecans), barley, rye, split peas, spinach, etc.
Zinc	Oysters, red meat, nuts, eggs, etc.
Chromium	Brewer's yeast, beef liver, wheat.
Selenium	Butter, oily fish that is smoked, wheat, nuts.
Iodine	Seafood, liver, nuts, etc.
Nickel	Soyfoods, beans, lentils, oats, etc.
Molybdenum	Lentils, liver, peas, cauliflower, wheat, etc.
Vanadium	Buckwheat, soy, parsley, eggs, corn, etc.

Highlighting Problems of Nutrient Depletion in Food

Intensive farming in many countries has tended to deplete soils of many nutrients, but this depletion is a particular problem when it comes to minerals and trace elements. Whilst it is relatively easy to measure dietary intakes of carbohydrates, fats, the assessment of dietary mineral intake from food tables (used by dieticians or nutritionists) are fraught with errors. These errors are due to the wide variation in trace element content of foods. Analyses of different plants from different growing areas in the same general location can show major variations in trace element content. Other factors determine the nutrient content of fruit and vegetables. These factors include the strain of plant, climatic conditions, maturity of the plant, etc.

There as some well-described examples of this phenomenon of variable nutrient content of plants. For example, the content of manganese is highly variable from plant to plant even within the same field of growth. In addition, it is well known that immature legumes, e.g. soybeans, have major variations in phytochemical contents depending on their degree of maturity.

Some alarming trends have been noted in the mineral and element content of major staples in Western diets. It would appear that the mineral content of many grains may be steadily decreasing. This situation has resulted largely from changing soil characteristics and fertilizer treatments. Horticultural and botanical studies confirm these problems with mineral depletions of soil. For example, careful studies of the chemical content of vegetables grown in gardens in Western Canada have shown quite major variations in copper, zinc, lead and molydenum content. There has been a tendency to ignore this circumstance of mineral depletion during crop production. The dangers of depletion of soils have been *"cast off"* by statements that plants will not grow without minerals. This is not true. Botanists have catalogued the symptoms and signs of *"sick plants"* that grow under mineral deprived circumstances. There are types of plants that may grow in abundance in the presence of certain mineral deficiencies. For these reasons, many individuals have sought a predictable intake of vital minerals in the form of dietary supplements, such as coral calcium. After all, the trace mineral content of fruit and vegetables reflects the mineral content of the soil in which they were grown. Whilst we browbeat ourselves about eating more fruit and vegetables, we tend to forget the modern trend for plants to be depleted of minerals and trace elements.

The Concept of Marginal Deficiency of Trace Elements

There has been a concern expressed among nutritionists for many years about our lack of understanding of *"marginal"* dietary deficiencies of trace elements. In simple terms, marginal deficiency refers to a state where minerals are present in the diet in inefficient quantities. It may come as a shock to some when I propose that three quarters of all people in the U.S. and Canada may have marginal deficiency of one or more minerals or trace elements. It has been suggested repeatedly that much more research is required on trace element deficiencies and their effects on health. In contrast, there has been a concerted effort to warn about the dangers of mineral excess, even though toxicities from minerals usually occur in special circumstances (e.g. calcium or magnesium excess in the presence of renal failure is dangerous.) In fact, the lack of knowledge about the importance of trace minerals in nutrition has made the setting of recommended daily intakes very difficult. In many cases, these recommended intakes are best guesses, and in most cases they are ridiculously low.

More Is Not Necessarily Better In Some Cases

Throughout this book, I have stressed the importance of abundant mineral intake and whilst this results in health and well being for the vast majority of people, there are circumstances in which excesses of nutrient minerals can cause problems. These circumstances usually result from the presence of severe and established diseases such as renal failure or severe metabolic disorders where imbalance of minerals exists in a critical manner, e.g. people with severe heart disease taking drugs that alter mineral status.

In my book entitled, *The Calcium Factor*, I point to evidence that toxicities of mineral nutrients have been overemphasized in some areas of medical literature. In addition, I present evidence that similar concerns about excess in vitamin intake may have been on occasion over-inflated. However, I do advise that anyone with doubts about their own health are best advised to seek the assistance of a skilled health care practitioner, before they attempt to self-medicate.

I emphasize that the form in which people may take dietary supplements can result in adverse outcomes. For example, some studies have shown that rapidly absorbed, ionized forms of calcium can upset calcium balance in a rapid manner causing unpleasant symptoms. One real advantage of coral calcium is its tendency to not result in rapid swings of high (hypercalcemia) or low (hypocalcemia) blood calcium. One important research study has been published recently in a book, written in Japanese and entitled, *Warning! Calcium Deficiency* (Shundaiyoyosha Publishing Co., Tokyo, Japan, 1999). This book, based on a massive study done in Japan, confirms the advantages of coral calcium from Okinawa as a safe dietary supplement.

The Ideal Properties of Coral Calcium As A Supplement

In the book, *Warning! Calcium Deficiency*, S. Kawamura and T. Taniuchi reported that a 30-year study with 20,000 case histories of over 40 over-the-counter calcium products, found that those people taking liquid ionized calcium were suffering from acute hypercalcemia as evidenced by such symptoms as muscle weakness, polyuria, dehydration, thirst, anorexia, vomiting and constipation, followed by stupor, coma, and azotemia in severe cases. Due to the rapid increase of calcium in the blood, the kidneys will attempt to reduce the excess calcium by excreting it in urine. This abrupt lowering of calcium may result in *"hypocalcemia"* causing muscle cramps, tetany, convulsions, respiratory distress, diplopia, abdominal cramps and serious metabolic disorders. However, the authors discovered that in over 30 years of study, none of the hyper/hypocalcemic symptoms occurred with those in the 20,000 who ingested coral calcium or other marine calcium products.

Richard Wood, Chief of the Mineral Bioavailability Laboratory at the Human Research Center at Tufts University in Boston, reports on 30 cases of calcium toxicity *"from taking too much calcium over time."* The symptoms were fatigue, dizziness, and soft tissue calcification. Of course, this is a very small group, and the hormone calcitonin, produced as a result of the sun striking the pituitary gland, could have prevented their hypercalcemia. Thus, the problem was not excess calcium consumption, but rather, lack of exposure to sunshine. Also, according to this previously discussed massive Japanese study, had the thirty individuals been taking coral calcium, they would have never had problems with hypercalcemia, regardless of exposure to sunshine.

Minerals and the Elderly

There are many gaps in our knowledge about mineral

and trace element deficiencies in the elderly. The variability of mineral status in older people is considerable. Malnutrition in the elderly has many contributory causes including poor health, aging of digestive organs with compromised function and economic or social problems.

Some studies show that poor nutrition is not confined to the elderly living at home, it is quite common in institutionalized elderly people, even those in hospitals. Much knowledge on the body status of minerals and elements and their requirements by the elderly is incomplete. Medical scientists have tended to use information that has been collected in young adults and they have attempted to apply this to the elderly.

It is likely that mineral and trace element deficiency in the elderly is a significant problem or risk because a tendency for a decline in total food intake and alterations in the digestive and absorptive efficiency of the gastrointestinal tract. Soil depletion of minerals contributes to nutrient reductions of plants, which are also processed in ways that can reduce their nutrient metal content. Many Western diets rely heavily on cereal intakes and the adequacy of copper and zinc intake is a concern with cereal dependent diets.

There is much debate about toxicity of certain elements with advancing age. Particular concerns have been expressed about accumulations of fluorine, lead and cadmium, especially in industrial societies. Whilst lead and fluorine are deposited in bones, cadmium may locate in the kidneys and cause impairments of kidney function.

There are a few essential elements that decline in human tissues as a consequence of aging. The importance of calcium, magnesium and zinc depletion are well-defined, but less attention has been paid to important and significant reductions of tissue levels of chromium and silicon. Considerable information exists in relationship to the biological activity of chromium compared with silicon. Medical studies have shown that chromium levels decline with age in the body tissues of people in industrialized societies. There seems to be a special relationship between chromium and control of blood glucose.

It has been noted that the livers of individuals with diabetes mellitus have low levels of chromium and it is known that this element is an important factor in the action of insulin. Western communities have an epidemic of maturity onset type diabetes, which is related to obesity. In fact, the estimates of its occurrence may be as high as 15 percent of the entire adult population and I believe that mineral deficiency, especially chromium is related to this problem.

Silicon is essential for bone, joint and skin health. Animal studies show gross deformities of bones if low silicon diets are fed. It appears that without silicon normal connective tissue and cartilage does not form in the body. In addition, silicon seems to decline in the walls of arterial blood vessels with age and this situation contributes to hardening of the arteries that commonly cause heart disease, poor circulation, organic brain disease and stroke in older people. Certain derivates of silicon e.g. asbestos are quite hazardous to health and much more research is required to define silicon's role in body functions.

It is well recognized that the ability to absorb calcium is impaired with age and the elderly adapt poorly to low calcium intake in their diet by accelerated bone loss. Several factors account for this problem, in addition to calcium deficiency. These include lack of vitamin D in the diet and reduction of vitamin D synthesis in the skin of old people, especially if they do not expose themselves to sunlight.

One factor that has been overstressed as a cause of calcium deficiency in the elderly is a reduction of gastric acid that may occur with advancing years. A lot of this problem is caused by the avoidance of table salt which is crucial in the manufacture of hydrochloric acid. A recent study by the Albert Einstein Institute of Medicine showed that when the elderly doubled their salt intake, the incidence of heart disease was reduced by 400 percent. Fortunately, ionic and especially chelated forms of calcium are well-absorbed and calcium is found in this form in coral calcium. The Japanese experiments that show efficient absorption of calcium from coral calcium reinforce the ideal nature of coral calcium as a supplement to help avoid problems with calcium deficiency that are common in the nature adult and the elderly.

A discussion of the health status of mature adults and its relationship with nutritional status is very important. Certain disorders occur with aging and many are amenable to partial or complete correction of mineral status. Table 25 gives some examples of minerals/trace elements and disorders of aging.

Table 25
Some Examples of Age-Related Disorder and The Influence of Toxic and Nutrient Elements

Age Related Disorder

Comment	Comment
Bone health, cardiac health, cancer.	Calcium and magnesium play a key role in bone health, potential for maintenance of cardiovascular health, and calcium is protective against certain types of cancer. Selenium protects against heart disease.
Diminished taste and smell in the elderly	Copper deficiency can cause loss of taste and smell.
Diabetes mellitus	Zinc and chromium are necessary for insulin production and actions.
Mental disorders	Zinc deficiency may precipitate depression.
Alzheimer's disease	Aluminum and silicon are deposited in the brain. Altered calcium status present in dementias.

Chronic Fatigue Syndrome and Minerals

Chronic fatigue syndrome (CFS) is a poorly characterized disorder. Some hidebound physicians even deny its existence, but the people who suffer the debilitating effects of this disease strongly disagree! Most healthcare givers recognize the varied symptom complex of CFS but few have successful experiences in treating this disorder. Ill health with CFS includes weakness, excessive tiredness, joint symptoms, depression, muscle pain and other debilities. There are many theories to explain the cause of CFS, which is most often believed to be a chronic viral disorder.

Whilst the cause of CFS remains uncertain, I have no doubts that mineral and trace element imbalances play a major role in the manifestations of CFS. It should be noted, that lack of oxygen causes fatigue, and the acidosis resulting from mineral deficiency results in a loss of oxygen. Also, many individuals have claimed positive benefits from mineral supplements in this disorder and relief has been noted frequently in people with CFS who take coral calcium. The disorder of CFS is never diagnosed in Okinawa!

Many nutritionists and physicians (both conventional and *"alternative"*) have used vitamin and mineral supplements with benefit in CFS. In the best-selling, informative book entitled, *Chronic Fatigue Syndrome – The Hidden Epidemic* (Harper Perennial, NY, NY, 1992), J. Stoff M.D. and C. Pellegrino Ph.D outline the importance of calcium and magnesium (with other elements) in the effective treatment of CFS. These authors describe the important actions of magnesium with vitamin B complex in supporting liver function and calcium with magnesium can deal with many symptoms of CFS, especially troublesome insomnia that plagues some sufferers of CFS. With CFS, immune function is impaired and several elements, especially zinc and magnesium, are required to promote healthy immune function.

Drs. Stoff and Pellegrino emphasize the problems that we face with mineral depletion of vegetables. They state, *"Vegetables in your local supermarket are not only twice as big and twice as expensive as those grown before the 'green revolution' (the widespread use of synthetic fertilizers), but you'll probably have to eat twice as many to get the same nutritional value."* Mineral supplements are a mainstay of nutritional advice for people with CFS. Later, one will be able to read some of the personal, positive experiences of the use of coral calcium in CFS and its variants of plain old tiredness!

Hair Analysis For Minerals

The whole issue of detecting marginal deficiency of minerals and trace elements is quite problematic. Simple tests have not emerged that permit an easy identification of mineral deficiencies. For more than fifty years scientists have been developing ways of measuring trace elements and minerals in body tissues. One controversial, but increasingly accepted measurement technique, is the assessment of trace minerals in samples of hair. The hair follicle has a distinct anatomy and the growth of hair provides clues to the environmental history and development of a person over a period of time. The same is true about nails and teeth.

The value of elemental analysis of hair is hotly debated between conventional and alternative medicine. In the technique of hair analysis for trace mineral assessment, a clump of hair is taken from close to the scalp, treated with acid and subjected to chemical analysis of its content of elements. There are problems in the interpretation of hair analyses. Hair composition is changed by external agents (e.g. dyes, shampoos, environmental pollutants) and there are few laboratories in the US that have developed standards with which to compare individual results. Exceptions are the labs of Great Smokies Diagnostic Laboratories in Asheville, NC and Doctors Data Inc. in Chicago.

Whilst hair analysis for trace elements may be valuable in some circumstances, there is no evidence that it can predict vitamin or the status other nutrients. The value of hair analysis is related to the skill exercised in interpreting the significance of the findings. The levels of minerals in hair do not bear a simple relationship to body stores. For example high zinc, calcium and magnesium levels in hair may signal a deficiency of these elements, not an excess, as the body is using the hair to shed these minerals. Whilst potentially valuable, hair analysis as a guide to mineral needs or status is not always accurate.

Marginal Mineral Deficiencies Effect Health

Most accounts of mineral or trace element deficiencies in the medical literature focus on overt, severe deficiencies and their consequences. In fact, the recognition of trace mineral deficiencies has been a relatively recent phenomenon in medicine. The history of the discovery of mineral deficiencies is a *"hotch potch"* of discoveries. For example, forty years ago, certain forms of heart disease were recognized in a remote area of China as a consequence of selenium deficiency and dwarfism was identified in the Middle East in the 1970s as a consequence of zinc deficiency. Some of the most important discoveries on elemental deficiencies were made on patients who were receiving intravenous feedings in hospitals. In these circumstances, certain trace element deficiencies were found to result in serious disease. The detection of toxicities from excesses of trace elements was made often as a consequence of isolated geographic events e.g. selenium toxicity in California causing hair loss, liver disease and gastrointestinal disorders etc.

When discussions occur about appropriate intakes of minerals there must be a clear distinction between an amount to prevent overt deficiencies and an amount to provide levels that are optimal for the normal functioning of body chemistry. Thus, the definition of *"marginal"* deficiency has not reached a consensus opinion. In order to overcome this situation, scientists have proposed definitions for trace element intake that involve the concept of an estimated safe and adequate daily dietary intake or ESADDI for short. Thus, the recommendations for optimal intakes of minerals are far from an exact science and they tend to be revised upwards as the importance of marginal deficiencies of minerals become more obvious.

One might question the need for such a detailed debate, but I believe that marginal mineral deficiency is a major, overlooked, public health concern in Western society. There has been a notable lack of research to relate marginal mineral deficiencies to health problems. So vital and extensive is humankind's need for mineral intake, that deficiencies may play a role in almost all common diseases, but this role lacks clear definition.

Progress has been made in the area of calcium, magnesium and zinc research. For example, growth retardation in children is well associated with marginal zinc intake and calcium deficiency is associated with osteoporosis in an unquestionable manner. However, the role of marginal intake of calcium and magnesium as a cause of heart disease or cancer has taken second place to other nutritional theories of causation.

Animal or human experiments help to elucidate the negative health outcome of mineral deficiencies, but these studies are handicapped by a focus on one single micronutrient (trace element) deficiency. It is well recognized that trace elements function by interacting with each other and with other molecules in the body. Examples of this phenomenon abound. For example, excess zinc or iron intake can block the absorption of other elements e.g. zinc and copper. This makes the circumstances more complicated in estimating ideal mineral intakes in diets.

The distinguished nutritionist Richard A. Passwater Ph.D. has emphasized that trace mineral balance is essential in cancer and disease prevention (*Cancer Prevention and Nutritional Therapies,* Keats Publishing Inc., 1983). I agree with Dr. Passwater that trace minerals play a major role in the prevention of breast, colon and prostate cancer. Although studies have been at variance in some cases, largely due to flaws in scientific methods, it is known that copper deficiency predisposes to cancer, as does zinc and calcium deficiency. The mechanism whereby these minerals exert these effects is probably related to their positive effects on antioxidant enzymes. In particular, the trace minerals copper, manganese and zinc are part of the body's important antioxidant enzyme called superoxide dismutase (SOD). Antioxidants function to stop oxidative stress to tissues that is caused by free radical damage.

Whilst we know that trace elements function by a complex series of *"competitions and balances,"* the simplest and most effective approach that we have is to supply trace elements and minerals in steady amounts. Overall, the body has a tolerance to many minerals, so that in most circumstances mineral supplements are quite safe. The abundant mineral supply in Okinawa and in other areas of the world seems to attest to general safety and positive health consequences of abundant mineral intake in the diet.

When Are Minerals Dangerous?

Relatively large doses of common essential minerals such as iron have potentially serious consequences. It should be noted that relatively large doses of anything and everything can be toxic, including water (drowning). Large doses of iron can cause poisoning especially in children and excessive iron intake make cause oxidative stress on tissues, while doses too small can result in serious detrimental health consequences. Excessive zinc can diminish immune function whereas zinc deficiency causes major impairment of immunity. The fact is that the population of Western communities has a much greater risk of deficiencies of most nutrient minerals and trace elements than any risk of excesses. It should also be remembered once again that populations, such as the Hunzas, who are virtually disease-free, consume large amounts of the crucial minerals, such as 100 times the RDA of calcium, with virtually no toxic side effects other than good health.

Coral Calcium at Work

Having reviewed the potential mechanisms of action of coral calcium with its rich mineral and trace element content, the real issues pertain to its effects at restoring health. In common with other beneficial nutraceuticals that have been used with years' precedence of safety and effectiveness, there have been no controlled clinical trials of coral calcium in specific disease treatment.

This common status of affairs in complementary medicine or nutritional practice presents limitations in making claims about efficacy in disease treatment. However, the *"proof of pudding"* is in the result. In this section of the book, I share just a few of the many thousands of testimonials that I have received or witnessed on the use of coral calcium for health. The statements and clinical vignettes speak for themselves!

CHAPTER 11

Testimonials

Scientifically, testimonials are considered as hearsay and are inadmissible. The same is true in our courts. However, when the number of testimonials becomes significant, so does the content of the testimonies. Coral calcium has a track record of well over 600 years, with testimonies about health benefits from the very beginning. It was these testimonies that induced the Spanish explorers 480 years ago to fill up their ship holds with the coral calcium and to return to Europe where the testimonies continued, and have done so to this very day. Japan, China, Russia, Sweden, France and England have tens of millions of people taking coral calcium daily with reportedly millions of testimonials. Although many scientists recognize the limitations of anecdotal reports, the sheer numbers of reports on coral has become a scientific factor. Readers are not advised to self-medicate, but rather, take this new scientific information to discuss with their doctors, and to try to convince their doctors to join in 21st century medicine, preventive medicine. Coral has only been in America for a few years, but already the testimonies are flooding in. Following are a few examples:

Testimonies:

1. Hi to everyone,
Just wanted to let you all know that I've been using the Coral Calcium, and it is definitely helping me. I am esp. excited over the fact that I am sleeping better. My usual night activity is ***frequent urination***, getting up 6 to 8 times in a 8 hour period to use the bathroom, plus I wake up in pain all through the night. Since the very first night, I slept at least 4 hours straight before I had to relieve my bladder, then I took another calcium (not sure if it was necessary at that point) and slept like a baby another 4 hours. It's wonderful. This happens every night now. I have had such a sleep deficit for so long. Now some more good news: I have less pain. Oh thank God! I have Fibromyalgia, and after years of disability due to such horrible, constant pain, a wheelchair, and a walker, I have hope of getting better, and I'm not so fatigued. To have any less pain is a miracle, and such a Blessing. Now if I can start exercising and lose weight I will be so forever grateful to this product, and to Donna. Exercising makes Fibromyalgia worse, plus I have a back problem, a foot problem, and very weak legs. But somehow I know I'm going to keep getting better. THANKS to Donna for sharing this info with me. I encourage you all to try it also. I've taken other calcium products, but never achieved these good results.

Bless you all, Joanie O.

2. Hello, my name is Conrad Sims, I am 29 years old and I live in Decatur, Ohio. I am athletic and consider myself to be in good health. A few months ago my neck began to get sore and then began to swell. I tried to ignore it, but it began to become painful. It was not long before the swelling was the size of a golf ball and my co-workers demanded that I see a doctor. It was diagnosed as *malignant cancer* and the doctor told me that it had to be removed surgically. He said there was no other way. I did not have health insurance for the surgery and I was terrified. A friend suggested I try coral calcium. I thought, "what's a little calcium going to do for me?" I was desperate so I started taking the coral and within a week the pain had subsided. After two weeks the size of the tumor was dramatically reduced, and after four weeks it appeared to be gone. I am back to my old self and feeling great.

God bless coral calcium, Conrad Sim. (March, 2001)

3. My name is Sue Ann Miller and I live in Akron, Ohio. I had been suffering for years with several diseases: *diabetes, Bells Palsy, carpel tunnel syndrome*, and I have had hip, knee and elbow replacements. I lived on drugs and was in constant pain. I could barely walk and could not climb stairs. Then my sister went to a talk by Mr. Barefoot and brought me some coral calcium. I was in such pain and was so desperate that I would try anything. In just a few weeks the pain went away. A few weeks later and I returned to full mobility as my swelling went down and my hands straightened out. A few weeks more and I could bend over, touch my toes and run up stairs. I have gotten my life back. The coral was magic and I thank God for the coral and Bob Barefoot.

I love you all, Sue Ann Miller, Ohio.

4. My name is Allen Jensen and I have battled *high blood pressure* for years and have been diagnosed with diabetes for three years. Medication has helped me more or less keep both "in check," but has done nothing to lower either the blood pressure or my blood sugar level. Then, in October 1997, I was diagnosed with Guillain-Barre Syndrome, a neurological disorder in which the nerves are destroyed by a "glitch" in the body's immune system. I lost a great deal of strength and dexterity in my hands, arms and legs. My active lifestyle of riding horses and a 30-year career as a telephone installer/repair technician ended with no choice but to take early disability retirement. In mid May 2000, I began taking coral calcium. Blood work showed a drastic improvement from tests in November 1999. My triglycerides improved from 1074 to 510, cholesterol from 380 to 210, and my blood sugar from 284 to 168. My doctor told me to "keep doing whatever you're doing." With daily use of the coral calcium I am confident that I will eventually be able to discontinue all of my medications. Coral calcium has virtually given me back the life I was beginning to believe I would not be able to enjoy again.

Allen Jenson, Breckenridge, Texas.

5.   My name is Donna Crow and I am struggling to recover from *Chronic fatigue syndrome* which struck me severely 12 years ago. One of the problems with CFS victims, as I am sure you know, is that we have problems absorbing and/or using minerals. As a result we often have insomnia, and heart palpitations.

A friend told me about coral calcium. She sent me a tape by Dr. Robert Barefoot. I was skeptical because someone else had sent me coral calcium that came in little tea bags and I had tried it with no noticeable benefit. But I value this friend's nutritional advise and out of honor for our friendship I listened to the tape. It was so educational.

It opened up for me, a whole new understanding of the need for calcium in the body. I loved the information and was determined to try some.

I got my first bottle and opened a cap and dumped it in my mouth since I seem to absorb better when I do that and within two minutes I felt the most amazing things in my body. Peace would be the best word to describe it. And from that day on I never have had the stress in my chest I had, had for 12 years prior. And my digestion is wonderful now; no acid reflux anymore. And I have NO heart palpitations at all.

This product is more wonderful to me than I can say. Unless you have had constant heart stress and other calcium/magnesium related problems long term, you cannot imagine how wonderful it is to go through a day without those problems. It is like getting out of prison.

I have all my friends and family on this stuff and they ALL love it for various reasons. That is the beauty of getting your mineral needs met. Your body will use them to do the unique repairs that you need. The body is so smart. If you give it the tools to work with it will literally work wonders for you. Thank you for a product that has been like a miracle for me.

Donna Crow, Newport, Or.

6.   Hi, my name is Dorothy Boyer and I will be 80 years old in June 2001. I have had *problems at night time with my legs.* They get nervous feeling and I have to get up and stomp around the room to get it to stop and then retire again. It is quite tiring to have to do this every night. My

daughter has tried to help me with many kinds of calcium and magnesium products, some quite expensive and none gave relief. Then she found Robert Barefoot's coral calcium and said, "Try this." And the very first night I slept through the night without any leg problems. That was several months ago and I haven't had any nighttime leg problems since starting the coral calcium.

Also I am very happy because I feel like I can think again. I have been very active mentally all my life and just in the last year I started to have trouble concentrating and staying focused. After just a few days on this coral calcium I felt like I could think again. I am very happy about that.

The biggest thing though is that I have a congestive enlarged heart and it doesn't take much for me to get a really rapid heartbeat. Just putting on a blouse in the morning would cause my heart to race and I would have to sit on the side of the bed and just calmly breath until it passed. From the first day I took coral calcium I have not had that again and that is the thing I am most happy about. It was very scary and it is nice to not be afraid every day.

Sincerely,
Dorothy Boyer, Newport, Oregon.

7.   With nothing to lose, we started giving our *crippled arthritic dog*, Bandit, 2 coral calcium capsules every day, figuring that if an average person takes two per day to fight serious illness, then Bandit, at about 43 pounds, should take two. She takes her capsules in peanut butter! That was July 1, 2000. Within just a day or two, she was eating again and walking out into the backyard and "using the facilities." Within a week she was walking normally. In

two weeks she would actually "trot" out to the backyard, get on and off the couch, and come upstairs. By the end of three weeks she was actually playing "wrestling" with our four-year-old dog, something she had not done in two years. Our veterinarian saw her and asked what we had done to create the "miracle." He bought some coral and said that he would be experimenting on some of his patients. By August, Bandit was like a new dog. She'll actually run now!

Bob Zacher, Memphis, Tennesee.

8. My name is Lisa Macintire and my *18-year-old cat,* "Tootsie," nine pounds started *limping* about two years ago and became very stiff-legged. She couldn't jump on things like the washer where she eats. She obviously had arthritis and was getting worse. About 2 months ago I started giving her 2 capsules of coral calcium every day, and in less than 2 weeks, she stopped limping. I kept giving her 1 capsule each day after that. In less than a month she started jumping and climbing all over the furniture. A check-up by the Vet showed her blood work, urine, etc. revealed no ill effects. The Vet's words were, "She's in perfect shape." The only side effect Tootsie suffered was "feeling GREAT." This coral calcium is truly a miracle.

Lisa Macintire, Memphis, Tennessee.

9. I was diagnosed with *Multiple Sclerosis* in 1978, and along with the disease came excruciating pain. In 1986 a pump was surgically installed in my abdomen, which put morphine into my spinal fluid 24 hour a day, and brought me modest relief. Last year, after 9 times in the hospital and 8 surgeries someone introduced me to colloidal minerals, which began to turn my life around. When I heard about *Coral Calcium* I thought, "How is a calcium product going to help me?" Well, I tried it June 24th, and it didn't take me long to realize that this was not the run of the mill calcium. About the first of July, I realized that I had no pain. For the first time in 19 years I had no pain and I could work 12 hours a day without stopping to lie down.

Earl Bailley, Ph.D, Doctor of Divinity, Ohio.

10. Your book did wonders for me. I had reached the point that *joint pain* was a part of my everyday life. Then, six weeks on coral calcium and I had become virtually pain free. Now, one year later, I feel better than I have in eight or nine years. Now my only problem is making my family and friends believe that being healthy can be so easy.

Rick Whedbee, Covington, Georgia.

11. My husband Mark had *painful heel spurs.* He was advised to have surgery. He began taking coral calcium, 6 per day, and within 2 months he almost was pain-free. Within 3 months, all of the pain was gone and the doctors have advised that he no longer needs surgery. Coral was a miracle as Mark's job has him working on his feet all day long.

Betty Gosda, Illinois.

12. My name is Patty and my husband was recently diagnosed with *prostate cancer*. My husband is 69 years old, 6'6", and works 12 to 14 hours every day from 5am to 5pm and later. Rather than expose himself to the horror of conventional treatment, he began taking coral calcium. After three weeks he had more x-rays and no cancer was found. Three weeks later, he went for a second opinion and had more extensive x-rays and once again, no cancer was found. Godbless coral calcium.

Patty, Ponca City, Oklahoma.

13. First of all, I want to start off by telling you about my brother. Mr. Barefoot, you have spoken with my father several times about him. He has *lung cancer*. When it was detected, he had four lesions on his lung, one was the size of a peach seed. My dad convinced my brother to take coral calcium. After 6 weeks when they ran another scan, 3 of the lesions were immeasurable, the big one had shrunk 60%. AMAZING !!!

Jeff Townsend, Kentucky.

14. I just wanted to give you an update on my father-in-law, J.W. Mitchell. As you know he was diagnosed with *bone cancer and cancer in the blood*. About 10 days ago he began your coral calcium program. His body went through detoxing for a day to a day and a half. He stayed in bed with the flu-like symptoms you mentioned, but he is doing better now. He went for a bone scan and blood work last Thursday and we received the results yesterday (this is about 9 to 10 days of your treatment). They now say "there is no cancer in the bones or in the blood." The hospice workers are in awe as well. The doctors now tell him that he may have a pinched nerve. He's a fighter and even more so now that he received the news from doctors at the VA that there's no more cancer in his bones. He is convinced that he is still alive as a direct result of your coral calcium program.

Peggy Mitchell, Batesville, AR.

15. Just want to take a moment to thank you for all your help. What coral calcium has done for me over a brief period is nothing short of profound. I can't remember any time in the last 29 years that I wasn't *in substantial pain...* that is until now. I have tried every pain remedy the orthodox medical community has in their arsenal, including narcotics, steroids, and anti-inflammatories, just to name a few. Most of them did a great job of messing with my head, a feeling I literally hate, but did very little for the pain. I know almost nothing about the science behind this majestic mineral, coral calcium, I only know that it works. I have more energy, more range of motion, and less pain than I ever thought possible ! I know that there was a time in my life that I was pain free, I just couldn't remember how it felt until now. There are no words I can think of to adequately explain how much better I feel or what it means to me. Thank you so very much!

Best Regards, Gary T. Schilling.

16. I heard about your program from a lady who attended your meeting in Twin Falls this summer. My husband has a *rare genetic disorder called Alpha I-Antitrypsin,* which is genetic emphysema that develops because the liver is not functioning properly, therefore, the lungs do not function properly either. He has been under a doctor's care for 9 years. After learning about your recommendations to help heal disease, my husband began taking the vitamins and the coral calcium and has been on the program for 7 weeks. He let go of his drugs and monthly prolastin infusion program. He is now very careful about what he eats. He feels better and better every day and has just let go of his inhaler. He has seen great improvement. I would love to speak to you and share this miracle unfolding before our very eyes. You are wonderful... thank you for your research and efforts.

Mary Wiggins.

17. I thank you for the confidence that you built for me. After being diagnosed with *melanoma* with no real hope for treatment if it were to reoccur, I felt devastated. My surgery was done at the Mayo Hospital in Rochester which is suppose to be "world-renowned for its advancements in medicine," but that can't mean advancements in reference to the treatment of cancer!! I now feel a sense of security for which I thank you. In a world of chaos and pain due to surgery, I felt that I was "drowning" in a sense, and thank you, thank you, thank you, from the bottom of my heart and the hearts of my precious family in Minnesota. I have given your information to anyone who has felt the perils of ill health and you are indeed held in high admiration for your work and devotion to healing mankind!! YES for CORAL CALCIUM!!!

Marcy in Minnesota.

18. I can't believe how different I feel after taking coral calcium. I lived with *constant pain in my heel* for months. I could not jog because I could just barely walk. After taking coral calcium for two months, the pain is gone. I am back jogging. I would not have done this if had not been for you.

Thank you very much, Russ Tomin

19. When one has been active all their life, it is impossible to understand the pain one suffers when the body is ravished by *rheumatoid arthritis.* Knowing that it was important to stay active, I enrolled in a fitness class. One of the activities involved lifting weights (20 pounds) with my legs. Due to the weakened condition of my legs, I tore a vital part of my knee. This sent me to the doctor and to physical therapy. When the pain did not go away, the doctor realized that the Rheumatoid Arthritis had taken over. I had been diagnosed 37 years prior with lymph edema which had caused fluid buildup in my legs. There was no known cure. The fluid must constantly be pumped out of my legs. This caused further damage and I no longer could have the fluid pumped out. I was in exacerbated pain now. Then I learned about coral calcium. Within two weeks I began to notice an appreciable decline in the arthritic pain. Within three months I became pain free and I am off my walker. Also the swelling had gone down in my mouth and I could use my dentures once again. Even my barber commented on how thick my hair had gotten. I am now "72 years young" after only 3 months on coral calcium. I can't wait to see what 3 years on coral calcium will accomplish. All I can say is, God bless all those who have made nutritional discoveries, especially coral calcium.

Willette Barbee, Plano, Texas.

20. The "Cancer Answer." The first week of March 2001, my stepfather was diagnosed with *leukemia*. They wanted to start chemotherapy right away. He asked for a day delay so he could start a nutritional program with coral calcium. In addition, Bob Barefoot recommended vitamin D and other minerals. On April 3, 2001 he went back to the doctors to run further tests on his condition. The doctors were amazed and totally baffled. They told him for reasons unexplained he doesn't need chemotherapy and that everything checked out normal. Hey folks, I thought Bob Barefoot had a screw loose when he claimed "coral calcium" could cure cancer. Turns out, he was right!

Jane and Sharon Gerding, Baker, LA.

21. My name is Susan Hedrik, age 49. I worked in a furniture factory carrying, stretching and cutting large rolls of cloth until it almost destroyed my body. I've had *back surgery* and suffered from a painful bone spur on my right thumb which two doctors told me would have to be removed by surgery. I also suffer from *arthritis* in my left leg. I was introduced to coral calcium and began taking it on January 27, 2001, and after four weeks "MY BONE SPUR WAS GONE!!!" I now can walk without a limp from the arthritis and no longer have to begin my mornings with a heating pad on my neck. For me, coral calcium is a "MIRACLE!!!"

Susan Hedrick, IR from Lincolnton, NC.

22. I have a 14 year and 6 month *Dachshund* named "Andrea" suffering from *arthritis in her hindquarters.* She couldn't walk without falling over. She was unable to jump on a bed or the couch, even with the help of a foot stool. I purchased coral calcium for Andrea and after five days she was becoming more active. After eight days she was jumping on the couch, begging for treats and running and playing. Andrea not only returned to normal activity, she also lost six pounds. Coral calcium also helped her teeth. Since she only has half of her teeth, I used to break her dog biscuit in half so she could chew it. Now, she chomps it down whole. As for myself, I have chronic arthritis in my lower spine. After seeing what coral calcium did for Andrea, I began using coral calcium myself. After 4 days I no longer had to take my prescription drug "Relafen," which costs over $3.00 per pill (I was taking 2 per day). I now am a firm believer in coral calcium as I have personally witnessed what it can do.

Jack Polhill from Lincolnton, NC.

23. I would like to confirm that the use of coral calcium has been beneficial to my health. My *knee replacements* are deferred and my golf swing has improved. I'll be 74 this summer and I trust this sophomoric feeling is not second childhood.

Eugene T. Hall, Calgary, Canada.

24. I am an osteopathic physician practicing osteopathic manipulation in the cranial field in South Central, PA. I have a patient who has suffered from severe *fibromyalgia* for the past several years. Recently she started taking coral calcium. This patient has improved dramatically. She has more flexibility and motion in her muscles and joints than she has in several years and she is nearly pain-free on many days. She has been able to discontinue a multitude of other medication, including chronic pain pills. The information in your books and tapes corresponds well to the science, the practical, the safe, the reasonable. I thank you for the time you have expended educating us.

Marianne Herr-Paul, D.O.

25. My mother, who has been on coral calcium for the past two months, paid a visit to her doctor to have her *cholesterol* retested. Her cholesterol had dropped 204 points and the doctor was amazed! She is now a believer in coral calcium. I thank God for you finding this product that is changing people's lives and giving their health back.

Cindy Metzger

26. My cousin Shirley had been diagnosed in May with *breast cancer and colon cancer.* She was scheduled for a double mastectomy and was also going to have her colon removed. You advised her to take the coral calcium and other nutrients and by July the breast cancer was gone and the colon cancer had shrunk. (Note: The October 1, 1998 issue of *Annuls of Internal Medicine.*)

Patti Hernandez, Oklahoma City, Oklahoma.

27. I am 62-years old and have always enjoyed good health. In July 1997 I was diagnosed with *prostate cancer.* The diagnosis was confirmed with a biopsy and an ultrasound. Two of six biopsies were positive with cancer. My doctors strongly urged me to take hormones and have my prostate removed. I thought about it but looked for alternative remedies. For six months I boiled Chinese herbs and did Qui Gong exercises and thought that this kept the cancer in abeyance. But in the spring of 1998 a second biopsy turned out to be similar to the first. "As a result of reading *The Calcium Factor* I received excellent treatment and eventually cured myself of prostate cancer." A third biopsy in July 1998 showed only one positive but reduced active cancer. I continued to take coral calcium and other supplements. A fourth biopsy in January 1999 showed that where the tumors had been, there was now only benign prostatic tissue. I had beaten the cancer. As a result I would strongly recommend that anyone suffering from cancer or similar debilitating diseases, should study Barefoot's book, *The Calcium Factor* and take responsibility for their own health. I have yet to find anyone who has written such well-reasoned and scientifically based material. I have been taking coral calcium for 3 years and it has saved my life.

David G. McLean, Chairman of the Board, Canadian National Railways.

28. In October 1996 I was diagnosed with *prostate cancer.* The diagnosis was confirmed by biopsy. In October of that year I started following Robert Barefoot's coral calcium regime. In July 1997 I had another prostate biopsy in which no evidence of malignancy was found. The regime outlined in the book *The Calcium Factor* improves the immune system to where the body can heal itself, without intrusive measures like surgery, chemotherapy or radiation.

S. Ross Johnson, Retired President of Prudential Insurance Company of America.

29. "I am a physician, President and Executive Medical Director of Health Insight, S.B.S. and Health Advocate Inc. in the state of Michigan. I have extensive credentials and honors that reach the White House and Heads of States in other countries. Mr. Robert Barefoot has worked over the past 20 years with many medical doctors and scientists across the United States and in other countries doing Orthomolecular Research on various diseases. The information has been culminated in the book, *The Calcium Factor,* which has been used technically as Bibles of Nutrition. Many people I know have thanked Mr. Barefoot for *both saving their lives and returning them to good health*. Mr. Barefoot is an amazing and extraordinary man who is on a 'great mission' for all mankind. I thank God for Robert Barefoot and thank God for coral calcium."

Liska M. Cooper, M.D., Detroit, Michigan.

30. "Mr. Barefoot has been, and continues to be, an advocate for health and natural healing through nutrition and knowledge. He has championed the cause of well over 440,000 American women and children who have been exposed to *the toxic effects of silicone implanted devices.* Mr. Barefoot, one of the rare silica chemists in the world, has delivered a message of hope to these suffering individuals, who didn't have any hope before, but are now arming themselves with the book *The Calcium Factor* and are spreading the word, especially about the miracle nutrient, coral calcium. His work with hundreds of scientists and medical doctors, researching diet, has elevated him to one of the top speakers on nutrition in the nation.

Jill M. Wood, President Idaho Breast Implant Information Group, Boise, Idaho.

31. I graduated from Harvard University in 1942 (BSc Chemistry) and worked as a Research Director and in corporate management, and have been awarded two patents. Mr. Barefoot has been highly influential in my survival of *prostate cancer*, with which I was diagnosed in the fall of 1991. Because of his detailed knowledge of biochemistry, he has much more penetrating knowledge of the relationship between disease and nutrition, a knowledge not available to many trained dieticians because of their lack of biochemical background. With his expertise, he has aided me in not only arresting the progression of my disease, cancer, through diet and nutrition with coral calcium, but also reversing it.

Philip Sharples, President Sharples Industries Inc. Tubac, Arizona.

32. I am a chemist and have been involved in product development, specifically nutritional supplements. I have written numerous articles and lectured throughout the United States on these products, especially coral calcium, and the benefits of utilizing alternative medicine and alternative medical products within the U.S. healthcare regimen. Over the past three years I have traveled and lectured with Mr. Barefoot on numerous occasions all over the United States. He is recognized as a world-class expert on calcium, especially coral calcium, and its nutritional benefits for the human body. I have personally seen Mr. Barefoot's information help a lot of people.

Alex Nobles, Executive Vice President, Benchmark USA Inc., Salt Lake.

33. One year ago my son Tim had major *back surgery.* Several disks had been crushed and three surgeries were performed. Four disks were removed, part of his hipbone was removed and ground to mix with a fusing material, then four cadaver kneecap bones were put into areas where the disks were removed. He has two titanium rods, two cross braces and eight screws in his spine. He started on coral calcium the day after the surgery. The first follow-up doctor's appointment showed that the fusion was doing great, exceeding the doctor's expectations. He said that this surgery was one of the toughest cases he has had. He said that he was amazed with the results, and told us to keep doing what we were doing. When Tim ran out of coral calcium for 3 or 4 days, he complained of severe back pain, which disappeared as soon as he went back on the coral calcium.

Billy J. Stein, Ponca City, Oklahoma.

34. The meeting that I had with you changed my life and how I think about my health. I am the person whose cousin's wife you helped. She took your coral calcium and minerals and she no longer has a *brain tumor.* My cousin's name is Gary Elias and his wife's name is Diane Elias. They live in Woodbury, Connecticut and they are both grateful because Diane's brain tumor pretty much dissolved and has not returned.

David Querim, Connecticut.

35. In November 1999 I was diagnosed with *prostate cancer.* My PSA was 244! On the way home, I listened to your audiotape. Talk about having the hand of God in your life! I knew in my heart that this is what I should do. Once I started, I never deviated from the plan. The results were amazing after only one month! My PSA had dropped to 25.5. By May my PSA was 4.6 and I had my doctor and specialists scratching their heads over my instant recovery. My doctor said that he never expected me to live past the end of January 2000. We also prayed and my doctor told me that "maybe the prayer worked" but it could not have been the calcium and supplements. Fortunately others have listened. My brother-in-law no longer has high blood pressure, ulcers, or indigestion. His sister-in-law no longer gets cramps in her legs and her arthritis is getting better. Her 5-year-old grandson, who suffered so much from leg cramps no longer, has pain or cramping and he can sleep all night long. These are just a few stories.

Bob Heinrich, Keremeos, British Columbia.

Afterword

Although most of the individuals taking coral calcium have a remarkable story to tell, not everyone has a story. On the other hand, not everyone was sick and to my knowledge, not one significant side effect has been recorded. This cannot be said of the vast majority of allopathic treatments (drugs and surgery) that are the mainstay of Western Medicine. This is because drugs kill while God's nutrients cure. Also coral calcium has the distinct advantage of being compatible with many other therapies. And it has helped many people providing a wholesome mineral support for many body functions.

I started this book by identifying coral calcium as one of the elixirs of life. Coral calcium has a 600-year documented history. Millions have benefited. No other natural nutrient mix has such a track record. After many years of personal research, we have been able to explain many, although not all, of the reasons for its health-giving potential. Coral calcium is begging to be studied in controlled clinical trials. This is the mandate of the FDA, which refuses to do so because coral is a natural substance and therefore cannot be patented. What makes this a crime is that coral calcium will one day, without FDA approval, cure the world.

Suggested Reading and References

- Anderson, J.J., Felson, D.T., *Factors Associated with Osteoarthritis of the Knee in the First National Health and Nutrition Examination Survey (HANES I).* : *Evidence for an association with over-weight, race and physical demands of work.* **AM J Epidemiol** 128:179, 1988.

- Bales C.W., Drezner M.K., Hoben K.P., *Eating Well Living Well with Osteoporosis:* Duke University Medical Centre. Viking, Penguin Books, Inc. NY, NY, 1996.

- Brown, S.E. **Better Bones, Better Body,** Keats Publishing, Inc. New Canaan, CT, 1996.

- Dawson-Hughes B., Jacques P., Shipp C. *Dietary Calcium Intake and Bone Loss from the Spine in Healthy Postmenopausal Women.* **Am J Clin Nutr** 46:685-687, 1987.

- Felson, D.T., Naimark, A., Anderson, J., *The Prevalence of Knee Osteoarthritis. The Framingham Study.* **Ann Intern Med** 109:18, 1988.

- Gaby, A.R., Wright, J.V., *Nutrients and Bone Health.* **Health World,** 1988, 29-31.

- Heaney, R.P. *Nutrition and risk for osteoporosis.* In: Marcus R., Feldman, D., Kelsey, J., (eds) **Osteoporosis.** Academic Press, San Diego, Ca, 483-505,1994.

- Heaney, R.P., *Nutritional factors in osteoporosis.* **Annu Rev Nutr** 13: 287- 316, 1993.

- Holt, S., Gagliardi, G., Fuerst, M., **The Shark Cartilage Alternative For Bone and Joint Health.** Keats Publishing, New Canaan, Connecticut, 1997.

- Howden, C.W., Saleeby, G., Holt, L., Holt, S., *Follow-up of patients with NSAID-related complicated peptic ulcer disease (CPUD).* **The American Journal of Gastroenterology** 86, 9:1313,1991.

- Howden, C.W., Holt, S., *Acid suppression as treatment for NSAID-related peptic ulcers.* **American Journal of Gastroenterology** 86(12):1720-2,1991.

- Kontessis, P., Jones, S., Dodds R., Trevisan, R., Nosadini, R., Fioretto, P., Borsato, M., Sacerdoti, D., Viberti, G., *Renal, metabolic and hormonal responses to ingestion of animal and vegetable proteins.* **Kidney Int** 38:136-144,1990.

- National Osteoporosis Foundation, *National Objectives for Disease Prevention and Health Promotion for the Year 2000.* National Osteoporosis Foundation, Washington D.C., 1988.

- Nevitt, M.C. *Epidemiology of Osteoporosis.* **Rheum Dis Clin of N Am** 20.3 535:559, 1994.

- Riggs, B.L., Melton, L.J., *The Worldwide problem of osteoporosis: Insights afforded by epidemiology,* bone 17(5) (Suppl.):505S-511S, November 1995.

- Saleeby, G., Howden, C.W., Holt, S., *Over the counter (OTC) non-steroidal anti-inflammatory drug (NSAID) uses may be an important determinant of complicated peptic ulcer disease (CPUD)*. **The American Journal of Gastroenterology** 86, 9:1375,1991.

- *Second International Symposium on the Role of Soy in Preventing and Treating Chronic Disease,* Brussels, Belgium, September 15-18, 1996 Program and Abstract Book; proceedings to be published in **J Coll Nutr** 1997-8.

- Strause, L., Saltman, P., Smith K., Andon, M., *The role of trace elements in bone metabolism.* In:Burckhardt, P., Heaney, R.P., (eds), **Nutritional Aspects of Osteoporosis,** Raven Press, New York, pp 223- 233, 1991.

- Vermeer, C., Jie K-S G., Knapen, M.H.J., *Role of vitamin K in bone metabolism.* **Annu Rev Nutr** 15:1-22, 1995.

Bibliography

Abbas F, Trapp R, Lai G, kolm P, Colliver J, Vasudeva R, Holt S. *Sequential observations of symptoms and gastroduodenal damage due to non steroidal anti-inflammatory drugs(NSAIDS)*. **American Journal of Gastroenterology,** 83, 9:1028, 1988.

Bloom BS. *Cross-national changes in the effects of peptic ulcer disease.* **Ann Intern Med.** 1991; 114:558-62.

Bloom BS. *Direct medical costs of disease and gastrointestinal side effects during treatment of arthritis.* **Am J Med.** 1988;84:20-4.

Gabriel SE, Jakkimainen L, Bombardier C. *Risk for serious gastrointestinal complications related to use of nonsteroidal anti-inflammatory drugs. A meta-analysis.* **Ann Intern Med.** 1991;448:787-96

Garcia Rodriguez LA, Walker AM, Perez Gutthann S *Nonsteroidal anti-inflammatory drugs and gastrointestinal hospitalization in Saskatchewan: a cohort study.* **Epidemiology.** 1992; 3:337-42.

Greene JM, Winickoff RN. *Cost-conscious prescribing of nonsteroidal anti-inflammatory drugs for adults with arthritis. A review and suggestions.* **Arch Intern Med.** 1992;152:1995-2002.

Griffin MR, piper JM, Daugherty JR, Snowden M, Ray WA.

Nonsteroidal anti-inflammatory drug use and increased risk for peptic ulcer disease in elderly persons. **Ann Intern Med.**1991;114:257-63.

Guess HA, West R, Strand LM, Helston D, Lydick EG, Bergman U, et al. *Fatal upper gastrointestinal hemorrage or perforation among users and non-users of nonsteroidal anti-inflammatory drugs in Saskatchewan, Canada, 1983.* **J Clin Epidemiol.** 1988; 41:35-45.

Henry DA, Johnston A, Dobson A, Duggan J. *Fatal peptic ulcer complications and the use of nonsteroidal anti-inflammatory drugs, aspirin and coticosteroids.* **Br Med J (Clin Red Ed).** 1987; 295:1227-9.

Henry D, Lim LL, Garcia Rodriguez LA, Perez Gutthann S, Carson JL, Savage R, et al. *Variability in risk of gastrointestinal complications with individual nonsteroidal anti-inflammatory drugs: results of a collaborative meta-analysis.* **BMJ.** 1996; 312:1563-6.

Hochberg MC. *Association of nonsteroidal anti-inflammatory drugs with upper gastrointestinal disease: epidemiologic and economic considerations.* **J. Rheumatol.** 1992;19:63-7.

Holt S, Irshad M, Howlen CW, Maneiro M. *Nonsteroidal anti-inflammatory drugs and lower gastrointestinal bleeding.* **Dig Dis Sci** 38:1619-1623, 1993.

Holt S, Saleeby G. *Gastric mucosal injury induced by anti-inflammatory drugs (NSAIDs).* **Southern Medical Journal** 84, 3:355-360,1991.

Holt L, Holt S, Saleeby G, Todd M. *Gastroduodenal injury from nonsteroidal anti-inflammatory drugs: risk management issues.* **Gastroenterology Nursing** 14(3): 124-126,1991.

Howden CW, Saleeby G, Holt L, Holt S. *Follow-up of patients with NSAID-related complicated peptic ulcer disease (CPUD).* **The American Journal of Gastroenterology.** 86, 9:1313,1991.

Howden CW, Holt S. *Acid suppression as treatment for NSAID related peptic ulcers.* **American Journal of Gastroenterology** 86:1720-2, 1991.

Irshad M, gopal A, Saleeby G, Holt S, Howden CW. *NSAID use as a conributory factor in lower GI tract bleeding.* **The American Journal of Gastroenterology** 86, 9:1312,1991.

Langman MJ, Weil J, Wainwright P, Lawson DH, Rawlins MD, Logan RF, et al. *Risks of bleeding peptic ulcer associated with individual, nonsteroidal anti-inflammatory drugs.* **Lancet.** 1994;343:1075-8.

Laporte JR, Carne X, Vidal X, Moreno V, Juan J. *Upper gastrointestinal bleeding in relation to previous use of analgesics and nonsteroidal anti-inflammatory drugs. Catalan Countries Study on Upper Gastrointestinal Bleeding,* **Lancet.** 1991;337:85-9.

Saleeby G, Howden CW, Holt S. *Over the counter (OTC) nonsteroidal anti-inflammatory drug (NSAID) use may be an important determinant of complicated peptic ulcer disease (CPUD)*. **The American Journal of Gastroenterology** 86, 9: 1375, 1991.

Saleeby G, Holt S. *Why do patients with life-threatening complications of peptic ulcer (PU) take nonsteroidal anti-inflammatory drugs (NSAID)?* **The American Journal of Gastroenterology** 85, 9:1294, 1990.

Saleeby G, Holt S. *An alarming association between nonsteroidal anti-inflammatory drug (NSAID) use and complicated peptic ulcer (PU)*. **The American Journal of Gastroenterology,** 85, 9:1294, 1990.

Saleeby G, Howden CW, Holt S. *Patient understanding of NSAIDs and ulcer complications: a need for improvement.* **Proceedings of the Annual Meeting of the British Society of Gastroenterology,** 1991.

Saleeby G, Holt S, Holt L, Eleazor P. *Pattern and prevalence of nonsteroidal anti-inflammatory drug use in elderly patients with complicated peptic ulcer disease.* **Clinical Research** 39, 2:594A, 1991.

Smalley WE, Ray WA, Daugherty JR, Griffin MR.*Non-steroidal anti-inflammatory drugs and the incidence of hospitalizations for peptic ulcer disease in elderly persons.* **Am J Epidemiol.** 1995;141:539-45.

Wong S, Gilrane T, Holt S. *Pattern and determinants of peptic ulcer and veterans administration endoscopic practice.* **The American Journal of Gastroenterology** 85, 9:1299, 1990.

References

1. National Osteoporosis Foundation, *National Objectives for Disease Prevention and Health Promotion for the Year 2000.* **National Osteoporosis Foundation,** Washington D.C., 1988.

2. Nevitt, M.C. *Epidemiology of Osteoporosis.* **Rheumatic Disease Clinics of North America** 20.3 535:559, 1994.

3. Felson, D.T., Naimark, A., Anderson, J., *The Prevalence of Knee Osteoarthritis. The Framingham Study.* **Ann Intern Med** 109:18, 1988.

4. Holt, S. *Soya for Health.* Mary Ann Liebert Inc., Larchmont, NY, 1996.

5. Theodosakis, J., Adderly, B., Fox, B., *The Arthritis Cure.* St Martins Press, NY, NY, 1997.

6. NIH, *Optimal Calcium Intake.* **National Institutes of Health** 12.4. 1-24, 1994.

7. Bales C.W., Drezner M.K., Hoben K.P., *Eating Well, Living Well with Osteoporosis:* Duke University Medical Centre Viking, Penguin Books Inc. NY, NY, 1996.

8. Anderson, J.J., Felson, D.T., *Factors Associated with Osteoarthritis of the Knee in the First National Health and Nutrition Examination Survey (HANES I). : Evidence for an association with overweight, race and*

physical demands of work. **AM J Epidemiol** 128:179, 1988.

9. *Second International Symposium on the Role of Soy in Preventing and Treating Chronic Disease,* Brussels, Belgium, September 15-18, 1996 Program and Abstract Book; proceedings to be published in J Coll Nutr 1997-8.

10. Dawson-Hughes B., Jacques P., Shipp C. *Dietary Calcium Intake and Bone Loss from the Spine in Healthy Postmenopausal Women.* **Am J Clin Nutr** 46:685-687, 1987.

12. Brown, S.E. *Better Bones, Better Body,* Keats Publishing Inc. New Canaan, CT, 1996.

13. Gaby, A.R., Wright, J.V., *Nutrients and Bone Health.* **Health World,** 1988, 29-31.

14. Holt, S., Likver, L., Muntyan, I. *The Vegetarian Way to a Healthy Urinary Tract.* **Alternative and Complimentary Therapies** - 10-15, May/June 1996.

15. Kontessis, P., Jones, S., Dodds R., Trevisan, R., Nosadini, R., Fioretto, P., Borsato, M., Sacerdoti, D., Viberti, G., *Renal, metabolic and hormonal responses to ingestion of animal and vegetable proteins.* **Kidney Int** 38:136-144,1990.

16. Heaney, R.P. *Nutrition and risk for osteoporosis.* In: Marcus R., Feldman, D., Kelsey, J., (eds) **Osteoporosis.** Academic Press, San Diego, CA, 483-505,1994.

17. Heaney, R.P., *Nutritional factors in osteoporosis.* **Annu Rev Nutr** 13:287- 316, 1993.

18. Strause, L., Saltman, P., Smith K., Andon, M., *The role of trace elements in bone metabolism.* In: Burckhardt, P., Heaney, R.P., (eds) **Nutritional Aspects of Osteoporosis,** Raven Press, New York, pp 223-233, 1991.

19. Vermeer, C., Jie K-S G., Knapen, M.H.J., *Role of vitamin K in bone metabolism.* **Annu Rev Nutr** 15: 1-22, 1995

20. *International Symposium on Soymilk and Cow's Milk.* Spring Meeting of Korea Soybean Society. **Korea Soybean Digest,** Vol. 14, No. 1, July 1997.

21. Theodosakis, J., Adderly, B., Fox, B., *The Arthritis Cure.* St Martins Press, NY, 1997.

22. Tamblyn, R., Berkson, L., Dauphinee, D., Gayton, D., Grad, R., Huang, A., Isaac, L., McLeod, P., Snell, L., *Unnecessary Prescribing of NSAIDs and the Management of NSAID-Related Gastropathy.* In **Medical Practice Annals of Internal Medicine,** Volume 127, No 6, 429-43,1997.

23. Holt, S., Saleeby, G., *Gastric mucosal injury induced by anti-inflammatory drugs (NSAIDS).* **Southern Medical Journal** 84, 3:335-360,1991.

24. Harris, W.H., *Total joint replacement.* **N Engl J Med** 297:650- 654, 1977.

25. Amadio, P.J. Jr, Cummings D.M., Amadio P., *Non-steroidal anti-inflammatory drugs; tailoring therapy to achieve results and avoid toxicity.* **Postgrad Med** 93:73, 1993.

26. Saleeby, G., Howden, C.W., Holt, S., *Over- the- counter (OTC) nonsteroidal anti-inflammatory drug (NSAID) uses may be an important determinant of complicated peptic ulcer disease (CPUD).* **The American Journal of Gastroenterology** 86, 9:1375,1991.

27. Howden, C.W., Saleeby, G., Holt, L., Holt, S., *Follow-up of patients with NSAID-related complicated peptic ulcer disease (CPUD).* **The American Journal of Gastroenterology** 86, 9:1313,1991

28. Saleeby, G., Howden, CW., Holt, S., *Patient understanding of NSAIDs and ulcer complications: a need for improvement.* **Proceedings of the Annual Meeting of the British Society of gastroenterology,** 1991.

29. Saleeby, G., Holt, S.,Holt, L., Eleazor P., *Pattern and prevalence of nonsteroidal anti-inflammatory drug use in elderly patients with complicated peptic ulcer disease.* **Clinical Research** 39, 2:594A, 1991.

30. Irshad, M., Gopal, A., Saleeby, G., Holt, S., Howden, C.W., *NSAID use as a contributory factor in lower GI tract bleeding.* **The American Journal of Gastroenterology** 86, 9:1312, 1991.

31. Holt, S., Irshad, M., Howlen, C.W., Maneiro, M., *Nonsteroidal anti-inflammatory drugs and lower*

gastrointestinal bleeding. **Dig Dis Sci** 8:1619-1623, 1993.

32. Holt, S., Howden, C.W., *Omeprazole; overview and opinion.* **Digestive Diseases and Sciences** 36(4): 385-93, 1991.

33. Howden, C.W., Holt, S., *Acid suppression as treatment for NSAID-related peptic ulcers.* **American Journal of Gastroenterology** 86(12):1720-2,1991.

34. Riggs, B.L., Melton, L.J., *The Worldwide problem of osteoporosis: Insights afforded by epidemiology,* **Bone** 17(5) (Suppl.):505S-51 1 S, November 1995.

35. Black, D.M. et.al. for the Fracture Intervention Trial Research Group: R*andomized trial of effect of alendronate on risk of fracture in women with existing vertebral fractures,* Lancet 348:1535-1541, December 7, 1996.

36. *Second International Symposium on the Role of Soy in Preventing and treating Chronic Disease,* Brussels, Belgium, September 15-18, 1996. Program and Abstract Book; proceedings to be published in **J Coll Nutr.** 1997-8.

37. Burke, G., *Phytoestrogens as an alternative to conventional hormone replacement therapy.* **Proceedings of the First World Conference on Nutrition in Medicine.** NY, NY, October 1997.

38. Staines, N.A., *Suppression of collagen induced arthritis by oral administration of type II collagen: Changes in immune and arthritsi responses mediated by active peripheral suppression.* **Autoimmunity;** 16:189-199 1993.

39. Brown, S.E., *Better Bones, Better Body.* Keats Publishing Inc., New Canaan, CT.1996.

40. Rovetta, G., *Galactosaminoglycuronoglycan Sulfate (Matrix) in Therapy of Tibiofibular Osteoarthritis of the Knee.* **Drugs in Experimental and Clinical research** 18(1):53-57,1991.

41. Pipitone, V.R., *Chondroprotection with Chondroitin Sulfate.* **Drugs in Experimental and Clinical Research** 18(1):53-57, 1991.

42. Oliviero, U., et al. *Effects of the Treatment with Matrix on Elderly People with Chronic Articular Degeneration.* **Drugs in Experimental and Clinical Research** 17(1):45-51,1991.

43. Mazieres, B., et al. *Le Chondroitin Sulfate Dayns le Traitement de la Gonarthrose et de la Coxarthrose.* **Rev. Rheum. Mal. Osteoartic** 59(7-8):466-472,1992.

44. Kerzberg, E.M. et al. *Combination of Glycosaminoglycans and Acetylsalicylic Acid in Knee Osteoarthrosis.* **Scandinavian Journal of Rheumatology** 16:377-380,1987.

45. Mueller-Fa,bender, H., et al., *Glucosamine Sulfate Compared to Ibuprofen in Osteoarthritis of the Knee.* **Osteoarthritis and Cartilage** 2:61- 69, 1994.

46. Crolle, G., D'Este, E., *Glucosamine Sulphate for the Management of Arthrosis: A Controlled Clinical Investigation.* **Current Medical Research and Opinion,** 7(2):104-109, 1980.

47. Dovanti, A., Bignamini, A.A., Rovati, A.L., *Therapeutic Activity of Oral Glucosamine Sulphate in Osteoarthrosis: A Placebo-Controlled Double-Blind Investigation.* Clinical Therapeutics 3(4):266-272,1980.

48. Pujalte, J.M., Lavore, E.P., Ylescupidez, F.R., *Double-blind Clinical Evaluation of Oral Glucosamine Sulphate in the Osteoarthrosis.* **Current Medical Research and Opinion** 7(2):110-114, 1980.

49. Vajaradul, Y., *Double-blind Clinical Evaluation of Intraarticular Glucosamine in Outpatients with Gonarthrosis.* Clinical Therapeutics 3(5):260+, 1980.

50. Crolle, G., D'Este, E., *Glucosamine Sulphate for the Management of Arthrosis: A Controlled Clinical Investigation.* **Current Medical Research and Opinion** 7(2):104-109, 1980.

51. Tapadinhas, M. J., Rivera, I.C., Bignamini, A.A., *Oral Glucosamine Sulphate in the Management of Arthrosis: Investigation in Portugal.* **Pharmatherapeutica** 3(3): 157-161, 1982.

52. Vaz, A.L., *Double-blind Clinical Evaluation of the Relative Efficacy of Ibuprofen and Glucosamine Sulphate in the Management of Osteoarthritis of the Knee in Out -patients.* **Current Medical Research and Opinion** 8(3):145-149, 1982.

53. Gaby, A.R., Wright, J.V., *Nutrients and Bone Health.* **Health World,** 1988, 29-31.

54. National Osteoporosis Foundation, *National Objectives for Disease Prevention and Health Promotion for the Year 2000.* **National Osteoporosis Foundation,** Washington D.C., 1988.

55. Ken Kaiser. *Television Interview on New York Cable Sports Channel 1,* May 21, 1997.

56. *Personal Interview with Mark Letendre.* Head Trainer. San Francisco Giants. Shea Stadium. August. 1997.

57. Erasmus, U., *Fats that Heal, Fats that Kill.* Alive Books Burnaby BC, Canada, 1993.

58. Murray, T.M., Beutler, J., *Understanding Fats and Oils.* Progressive Health Publishing, Encinitas, CA.1996.

59. Kremer, J.M., *Dietary fish oil and olive oil supplementation in patients with rheumatoid arthritis.* **Arthritis Rheum** 33:810-20. 1990.

60. Passwater, R.A., Fish Oil Update. Keats Publishing Inc., New Canaan, Connecticut, 1987.

61. Belluzzi, A., Brignola, C., Campieri, M., Pera, A., Boschi, S., Migoli, M., *Effect of an enteric-coated fish oil preparation on relapses in Crohn's disease.* **N Engl J Med** 1996, 334:1557-60.

Order Form

Web Site: "barefootscureamerica.com"
Toll Free 866-723-2551

Name:_____

Address:_____

_____

Country/Zip:_____

Phone Number:_____

Yes, I / We would like to order more copies of *Barefoot on Coral Calcium - An Elixir of Life* or *Let's Cure Humanity* or *The Calcium Factor* or *Death By Diet.*

Please send___copies of_____.

@ $24.95 US each ($27.00 Canadian)

for a total of $_____.___

Please allow a shipping and handling

charge of 5.00 US ($7.00 Canadian) per book: $_____.___

Arizona residents please add appropriate tax: $_____.___

Total enclosed: $_____.___

(Please check addition carefully; incorrect totals will be returned unfulfilled.)

Please allow 2 to 6 weeks for delivery.

A quantity discount schedule is available upon request.

Mail this order form (or a copy) along with a check for the total amount to:

Complete Fulfillment & Distribution
P.O. Box 71058 | Phoenix, AZ 85050-1058, USA